I Am More Than My Body

THE BODY NEUTRAL JOURNEY

BETHANY C. MEYERS

G. P. PUTNAM'S SONS
NEW YORK

PUTNAM
— EST. 1838 —

G. P. Putnam's Sons
Publishers Since 1838
An imprint of Penguin Random House LLC
penguinrandomhouse.com

Copyright © 2023 by Bethany C. Meyers

Library of Congress Control Number: 2023936709
ISBN 9780593544747

Printed in the United States of America
1st Printing

Book design by Alice C. Woodward

I Am More Than My Body

To the future. The youth of today, the children of tomorrow, the generations that follow. May you heal the wounds of your ancestors. May you value the contents more than the shell. May you find acceptance and respect both for yourself and others.

To my mom, my nieces, my daughter kicking in my womb. To my dad watching from up above, my spouse holding me close on earth, my future children I'm still waiting to meet. To every client who has shared their body, their perseverance, and their heart with me, you are my lifelong inspiration and forever motivation.

A Note on Language

The people directly interviewed in the book have each let me know how they would like to be identified and have had approval over their quotations. Any inconsistencies are therefore a reflection of the unique perspectives of the people who have so generously shared their stories with me. This book invites in the experiences of people of different races, sizes, shapes, ability, genders, and religions. The language used to describe identity has been read through by people from within those communities in the hope that the reading experience will be as inclusive and sensitive as possible.

Contents

The Journey Starts Here   1

Chapter 1: What Is Body Neutrality?   9

Chapter 2: Body Bias   47

Chapter 3: A Rebel with a Cause   71

Chapter 4: Childhood Stories   97

Chapter 5: Neutral Movement   123

Chapter 6: Let It Go   167

Do We Ever Really Get There?   197

The Body Neutral Toolbox   205

Acknowledgments   223

The Journey Starts Here

When I was young, I used to watch Nick at Nite religiously. I particularly loved *Bewitched* and *I Dream of Jeannie*, two 1960s sitcoms featuring glamorous, magical protagonists. I remember being convinced that I had supernatural powers too, I just hadn't learned my signature move yet. Samantha the witch would wiggle her nose and Jeannie would stack her arms and blink to access her genie gifts, so all I needed to do was find my own twitch. I would sit in my bedroom, make a wish, and then try a combination of tongue swirls, head nods, and finger taps—hoping to unlock some magical power. If you had walked in on me, I'm sure it would have been a funny sight. Of course, I never discovered my magic move. Like all of us, I've had to ask, work, and plan for the things I want in life, some of which have happened and some of which haven't. To me, the realization that the things we want don't happen magically—instead they take conscious effort and practice, but are nearly always worth it in the end—is reminiscent of the body neutral journey that we are about to embark upon together.

In short, body neutrality is the idea that each of us is more than our body, and our worth is not limited to our physical self. It is the practice of respecting our body despite the fact that we may feel differently about it on any given day—love, hate, and everything in between. When I was first learning about body neutrality, I remember having so many moments when I just wanted to get there already and proudly declare, "Here I am, meet *body neutral Bethany!*" But that wasn't how my journey went. I would have days when I felt awful about my body, when my old eating disorder mindset would creep in and shame would take over. I also had days when I would pretend to be so completely in love with my body—and that felt empty as well, like I was masking the shame with a lie. And then I would have days when I would slide into neutrality, experiencing neither deep love nor deep shame, but rather a gentle respect for my physical self while prioritizing my emotional self. Sometimes that felt liberating and sometimes it felt unsatisfying. I'm here to tell you that both of those feelings—and anything in between—are okay!

Perhaps you may be hoping to read this book and find your quick fix into body acceptance. Maybe you are looking for a fuss-free solution to every problem you're facing. The truth is, that's not how it works, and you should be wary of anyone who tells you otherwise. This book doesn't make lofty promises, like fitness companies selling New Year deals or health food providers coming out with a fancy superfood. It is not the answer, the truth, the way, or the life. It is, I hope, a guide to a new set of skills which might support you. I'm not saying that the ideas housed between its covers don't have the power to have a profound impact on your life. They have certainly made dramatic shifts in mine. But I want expectations to stay realistic: this is not a book of life hacks, or a quick fix, or a one-stop-shop solution. It is not a cure-all. Practicing body neutrality in a world that is extremely biased is hard work. It's going to take effort, time, and a whole lot of grace.

What this book will provide you with is clarity, and a potential way forward. It will encourage you to deconstruct a lot of narratives in your mind, peel back the layers of the world you have been raised in, and interrogate the foundations of your relationship with your body and beyond. It will introduce a framework to help you manage and navigate some of your feelings, and offer lots of tangible guidance, journaling questions, and suggestions, to help support you on this journey. There is even a toolbox of tips from everyone interviewed in the book on page 205, which is a collection of their and my top advice. A lot of times, body neutrality involves sitting in a gray space—a place in the middle that can be uncomfortable. I promise I will be there to hold your hand and heart as you take these important steps.

As a fitness teacher, I developed a method to create an inclusive space for movement, founded in curiosity and a willingness to experiment without sticking to a rigid idea of what "success" looks like. That philosophy is something I have worked to bring with me into this book, and I hope it's something you will feel as you read it. When I present practical advice, I have aimed to do so in a way that feels nonjudgmental. I also present a range of experts' views for you to explore and connect with. I want you to think about how these ideas might apply to you. And also how do they *not* apply to you? What are you interested in getting curious about, and simultaneously what are you not? Where in this book do our ideas and beliefs align, and where do they differ? Individual thinking is celebrated here! I encourage you to do what is right for you, and not simply what has been suggested. This means you may not agree with everything in this book and that's okay. You are you, I am me, and together we have so much to learn from each other. What I will say is that you should give yourself permission to take this book at your own pace. Many of these issues run deep in all of us, and I want you to give yourself grace as you struggle with them.

In my classes I aim to give everyone practical tools they can use when I'm not there as well as when we are together. This book explains concepts and ideas, but ultimately it is encouraging a practice that you can take off the page, apply to your life, and keep getting better at. While there will inevitably be times when you slip off-track or feel like you've failed, the learnings never leave you. Once your mind is opened to the possibility that a new way of interacting with your body exists, there isn't a way to row backward from that. And the framework presented in this book will become easier to reconnect with over time, even if you're out of practice. Body neutrality is a journey and it doesn't have to go in a straight line, because the ultimate aim is to arm yourself with a new skill set.

Now, before we go any further, it's important for me to highlight how I have only ever experienced the world in a body that has been accepted and invited into nearly every imaginable space. As a white, slim person, the way my body intersects with society is privileged to an extent that I will never be able to fully comprehend. I have never experienced the realities of living in a marginalized body, nor one that the general population deems unworthy. While I have recognized elements of the queer identity in the process of my own self-discovery, in many contexts I get to choose whether I let the world judge me by my differences.

For some of you reading this book, the idea that you could be neutral about your body when the world you live in has so much bias and systemic prejudice may feel impossible. I don't know what that feels like, because I haven't walked in your shoes. That is one of the reasons I have welcomed so many other voices in the pages ahead. Voices of people who have had hugely diverse experiences in the world, due to their bodies, abilities, and identities. They include fat folks, persons with disabilities, queer folks, and people of color. My deepest hope is that this book will embrace a wide variety of bodies, and help open the door to body neutrality and respectful acceptance for everyone. The conversations in this book are not just my voice, nor only the voices of those I've interviewed; they are also *your* voice.

As we get ready to jump in, I am reminded of another silly memory from my childhood. On my first morning of kindergarten, my teacher told the class that we were going to play a game with a special shoebox. The box had been decorated and a hole had been cut in the top, and everyone had to stick their hand inside the box, feel the object within, and guess what it was. When the box came to me, I couldn't put my hand in. I was so scared of what I imagined was inside: something awful and gooey, or a mouse that was going to run up my arm, or something that would hurt me. All the other kids in the class put their hands in and made their guesses, but I couldn't do it. At the end of the game, the teacher opened the box and revealed that it was . . . a marshmallow. Soft, squidgy, sweet, and totally harmless.

Leaping into anything new and unknown can feel terrifying, and you may find yourself freezing at something that others find easy to embrace. To this day I have a fear of sticking my hand into anything I cannot see. If something gets stuck in my kitchen sink, it's almost impossible for me to reach my hand in to get it out. We can learn the marshmallow lesson and acknowledge that we don't always need to be scared to jump in, but it still takes courage to try something new. And I recognize that is the case with body neutrality too. I think there is something that is a bit terrifying in letting go of your body in certain ways and not having it be the most important thing about you. It may always feel scary and it may always take some courage, but at the end of the day, it's still going to be a fluffy little marshmallow waiting for you.

CHAPTER 1

What Is Body Neutrality?

How it began

I remember the first time I heard the term "body neutrality." I had been writing an article for a well-known health and wellness website, and they emailed me to ask if I could swap out the term "body positivity" for "body neutrality." You'll soon find out that these two practices are completely distinct, but back then it was the first time I had heard of body neutrality, and it stopped me in my tracks. Not in a good way—I was mad. No, I was fuming! I felt betrayed; I had worked so hard to gain a positive mindset about my body after coming out of eating disorders and body dysmorphia, and now what? I was supposed to feel neutral about it? I felt as though body positivity was being undermined, perhaps even criticized, by this other, unfamiliar label.

Being the type who hates being difficult yet loves challenging the rules (hello, Gemini), I wrote a carefully crafted email back to the editor. Slathered with southern charm and a touch of "bless your heart," my underlying message basically asked: why the hell would anyone want to be neutral about their body? Then I strapped on my metaphorical boxing gloves while I waited for a reply. But the response surprised me. Floored me actually. And to this day, the line that sticks out from that email is this:

> It's more the idea that bodies are bodies, you are where you are, and that's okay. You love yourself as a person, not just as a body.

You love yourself as a person, not just as a body. My jaw dropped, tears sprang to my eyes, the boxing gloves melted off my hands. A spotlight shone above my head and I swear angels started singing "hallelujah." (Okay, maybe a slight exaggeration there.) It hit me at once: *I am more than my body.*

I began researching body neutrality, and every article, every definition, every personal account made me feel more and more at peace. I continued to learn more; I spoke about body neutrality with my community; and most importantly, I began to implement it in my recovery and my everyday life. I watched myself begin to find my neutral zone as I steered away from both extreme shame and a toxically positive mindset.

For me, finding body neutrality was accompanied by a sense of incredible relief—the likes of which I had never experienced before. To be honest with you, I am still on that journey, because "body neutral" isn't a destination you arrive at and then live happily ever after, but rather a place that every time you visit, you bring back a souvenir to help remind you of it. The more times you visit, the easier it is to get there.

But what *is* body neutrality, I hear you ask from the back. Is it a replacement for body positivity, like that editor originally suggested? Or is it something completely separate? I get where the body positive/body neutral confusion comes from, because in a way they have the same aim—self-acceptance—and that is a beautiful thing. But to break it down simply: I like to say that body neutrality is the practice of steering away from self-hate without the pressure of having to love our body. Within neutrality there will be some days when we love our body and some days when we hate it, and many days in between. But no matter how we feel about what is staring back at us in the mirror, we work to respect our body.

Body neutrality is not saying that you shouldn't have any feelings about your body or that you should never think about your body, or that your body doesn't matter. But it *is* saying that your body does not dictate your worth. You are more than a body, and your value as a person extends far beyond your physical presence.

To some this might sound like common sense, but the truth for so many of us is that it requires a revolutionary shift in both outlook and behavior. Why is that? In truth, it's a variety of factors—many of which we'll discuss and explore throughout this book—but there is one central binary that is at the heart of it. When you look at how our society currently talks about bodies, you can clearly see two poles between which the pendulum swings: body shame and toxic positivity.

The first pole: body shame

Body shame is heavily supported by diet culture, which is an insidious set of beliefs that worships exclusionary body and beauty standards—think flat stomach, long legs, perky butt, big lips, glossy hair, clear skin. It disempowers anyone and everyone who fails to meet these often unattainable goals. At its most extreme, diet culture is the social consensus that your appearance and body shape are more important than any other part of you—more important than your personality and character, achievements and contributions. And yes, even more important than your health. But it can also play out in smaller, more individual ways that also negatively impact your self-esteem and self-worth. For some, it is that voice at the back of your head whispering that you are not good enough unless you have the "perfect" body.

What's worse is that the beauty goalposts keep moving. During some eras, it was deemed desirable to have a curvaceous butt and hips, with a tiny little waist. A decade later, the butt was out and a string-bean, thin-hipped shape was in fashion. Then boobs were back. As I write this, today's version of the "perfect body" is a seemingly impossible combination of individual body parts jigsawed together.

Since we aren't inflatable dolls, it's pretty difficult to get an entirely new body shape every decade. And many of these fashionable body types are unrealistic for the vast majority outside of expensive cosmetic surgery. "I did Weight Watchers three times, the first at eleven years old, which had to be approved by a doctor," recalls Ally Duvall, a fat activist and body image program manager at Equip, a virtual care team for eating disorders. "I tried every fad diet, restricted and punished myself in every way possible. But I never achieved any of the results. I always blamed myself when my body weight didn't change drastically, and this ended up pushing me further and further into brutal eating disorders. I starved myself literally, but I also starved myself of life."

While the details may change, in the Western world— or in societies influenced by Western media—there is an emphasis on thinness, only possible for many through diets and frequent workouts. And that starts young. Today, girls as young as three show a preference for thinness; a sample of first through fourth graders showed that 41 percent wished they were thinner.

"Diet culture has dominated the vast majority of my life," says Alex Light, body confidence advocate and author of *You Are Not a Before Picture*. "Probably from the moment I became aware of my body, I became aware of the fact that it didn't look the way it should. It didn't fit the ideal or the standard that was being reflected back at me from a really young age. I started dieting around the age of eleven and spent the next thirteen years flitting from one diet to another. I fully believed the diet culture myths that I would only be lovable, desirable, worthy, and successful if I was thin."

Over the pandemic, I had a strong urge to indulge in things from my childhood. Childhood foods, childhood movies, childhood TV shows. I also started watching movies from the early 2000s that had been staples in my teens, and I found it shocking to see how eating disorders were glamorized. From very specific jokes about anorexia and disordered eating to applauding weight loss, it's no wonder I thought it was cool not to eat. And that's before we even discuss the prevalence of rail-thin actresses in every popular film of the time.

We are inundated with certain messages loudly and explicitly through the media—both traditional and digital—but also implicitly through hospitals, medical offices, schools, and public health providers. Carbs are bad, fat is bad, protein is good but only in combination with a low-fat food source. Eat intermittently, fast overnight, fast after 5pm—*is there a "right" time to eat?* Skip breakfast, don't you *dare* skip breakfast, try lemon water, drink protein shakes, cut out all sugar. Go running every day but running is bad for your joints, walk but that's not really a workout, lift weights but don't get too bulky, do squats for a bigger butt but don't beef up your thighs, get in 10,000 steps or else . . . *whoops*, turns out 7,000 is enough. Coffee is bad, coffee is good. Chocolate is bad, chocolate is good. Wait! Only *milk* chocolate is bad. Don't drink dairy milk. Drink soy milk. JK, we meant almond milk. Actually it's oat milk now.

Diet culture is like hundreds of contradictory voices screaming at you at once; at its extreme, eating and moving become so loaded with anxiety and expectation that we forget how to do either with ease. And what have humans been doing intuitively since the beginning of time? Eating and moving. We were born with these instincts.

Diet culture can also be quiet, however. Like many families, the women in mine were conditioned to feel shame toward their bodies; and while diet talk was never overt, it was always present. My grandmother, mom, and aunts would regularly discuss the desserts they shouldn't be eating or the weight they needed to lose before putting on a swimsuit. SlimFast and other nineties diet products invaded our household, and were seen as moral artifacts—a sign we were a health-conscious family. What we didn't know was that most of these products were filled with chemicals that caused more harm than good.

Why weight loss is not the answer

At the heart of diet culture is a lie. We are told that if we have enough willpower to keep up with a diet, we will lose weight and all our troubles will disappear. We will be happy, accept ourselves, find true love, gain more friends, be good at math, have organized junk drawers, climb Mount Everest! Okay, perhaps not all of those, but you get the idea: weight loss promises a lot of things. If only we can get to a certain weight or fit into a certain pair of jeans, then we will finally be at peace with our body. But that rarely happens. That could be because body ideals shift and suddenly that tiny butt and slim thighs you strove to achieve has fallen out of fashion. Or maybe because the sacrifices you've made to keep your body static prevent you from finding joy in life. Or perhaps because others simply don't care in the way you think they do.

Stephanie Yeboah, body image advocate and author of *Fattily Ever After*, shares an experience that highlights all of these empty promises: "When I was twenty-two, I underwent a dangerous fasting-based diet and ended up losing four stone [fifty-six pounds] over the course of four months. I had thought that if I were smaller, I'd get attention from guys, people would be nice to me, I would never get bullied and everything would be perfect. I had a birthday coming up and I wanted to go on a beach holiday, and I felt that to have a 'bikini body' I needed to look a certain way. I imagined that after losing all that weight, people were going to stop and stare and I would get flirted with. But none of that happened. I walked onto the beach in Barcelona, and nobody batted an eyelid. I made myself very sick for other people's validation, and I got no attention whatsoever. That was the moment I realized I needed to learn to love myself and my body. I was so tired of apologizing on behalf of my body as opposed to apologizing to my body for everything I had put it through."

Sometimes it seems like we would do anything for weight loss, no matter the cost. I've heard people refer to the "heartbreak diet" as a silver lining to a difficult breakup. What's next? The redundancy diet? The grief diet? The flu diet? Oh wait—that's a thing. There are many times in our lives when our bodies might fluctuate and we might gain or lose weight, several of which are connected to trauma and crisis. The glorification of the weight loss of these experiences is horrendous. A while ago, one of my friends was bemoaning the fact that she had gained weight. "Look at what I looked like last summer," she said, showing me old photos. "I was working out all the time and I looked great." My immediate response was to remind her what she had been going through at the time. After a difficult breakup she had been so low, she'd hardly been able to get out of bed. As she emerged from the fog, she started working out excessively even though she was barely eating. Looking at those pictures, she had forgotten all the unhappiness that went into being that size and was holding herself to an unsustainable standard.

Since healing from eating disorders, one of the things I value the most about my new life is that I get to experience eating with other people. Breaking bread represents how beautiful it is to sit and eat freely with friends. The ability to enjoy each other's company and share flavors, cultures, and customs is magical, and it's something I didn't realize I was missing. Food can be therapeutic. It can be a way to connect with other people and enjoy and experience life. How many of those experiences are we willing to lose in order to be thin?

I'm not ashamed of my past, but some of it is very difficult to discuss, especially when it comes to eating disorders and addiction. Some of the events in my life that you will read about in this book are extreme; many are mundane. Some might resonate immediately with you, while others might take some time to process. Either way, I hope they inspire you and help you reflect.

For many years, I looked like the embodiment of health—a poster child for the standards of diet culture. I had all the assets of what is deemed a "good body" by mainstream society. But I starved myself so much that whenever I did allow myself to eat—some grapes in between teaching classes—I would be violently sick because my body had gotten to a point where it could no longer stomach food. In contrast to how I was perceived by my clients, I was actually damaging my body in so many ways. When I think about that time in my life, it feels like the yarn was unraveling and making knots at the same time. I had a toxic relationship with my boss at work, an abusive relationship with my partner at home, an addiction to unprescribed amphetamines, eating disorders that had taken on a life of their own, and I had no idea how to get out. Everything was a mess.

No matter how much weight I lost, it was never enough. I was always able to find things wrong with my body. Have you ever heard the phrase "If you can't love yourself at a size 10 you won't love yourself at a size 4"? It's clichéd, but it's not wrong. Weight is surface-level; who you are underneath remains the same. Weight loss through shame, extreme restriction, and guilt does not a happy person make. Being in touch with your emotions, healing old trauma, practicing intuitive eating, exploring movement for joy . . . these things can dramatically change your outlook. Yes, they can lead to weight loss, but they can also lead to weight gain. I want to be explicit about this very early on: I'm not demonizing someone's weight changing, because bodies fluctuate. But I am asking us to look at the intent and the method, and explore if changing our physical self is truly serving us.

The second pole: toxic positivity

So, let's go back to the body talk pendulum (remember that?). If on the left side we have body shame fueled by diet culture, now I want to think about the other side: a toxic, twisted version of body positivity, which has distorted the admirable goals of a decades-old grassroots resistance movement and made us think that we must love every single thing about ourselves, at every single moment, with a fierce and unshakable passion. Someone recently described this toxic positivity movement as "shitting rainbows," and I half laughed, half cried at how accurate that was.

The origins of the body positive movement are revolutionary, and wildly important to the strides we've made in body acceptance. To be clear, body positivity is an incredible tool that has helped many people exist in this world. Body neutrality does not negate body positivity—they can work in tandem. But what I do want to explore is how toxic or fake positivity can be just as damaging as body shame.

The body positive movement has always sought to promote radical self-love and self-acceptance for your unique bodily form. Stretch marks? Gorgeous. Fat rolls? Magnificent. Body scarring? Truly individual. It campaigns for a wholehearted rejection of body shame and diet culture, because we are all beautiful exactly as we are right now. This book and the ideas of body neutrality build upon the work of the body positivity movement, which finds roots in the fat acceptance movement (encompassing fat pride, fat power, and fat liberation) which began in the late 1960s. Before it was used to sell you a deodorant, body positivity was best understood as a social movement focused on the acceptance of all bodies, regardless of size, shape, gender, race, or abilities. It has always sought to challenge beauty standards and social, medical, and cultural stigmas, and to help every person find self-love. Its history is enmeshed with radical social justice, feminism, the civil rights movement, and Black liberation, and was created by people in marginalized bodies (especially fat, Black, queer, and disabled bodies) for others living with similar prejudices.

"A lot has changed thanks to the body positive movement, and in particular there has been a massive increase in the choice and accessibility of clothing. Before 2010, there was virtually nothing you could wear if you were a fat woman who wanted to be part of youthful fashion. The clothing we had was very frumpy," recalls Stephanie. "But as soon as activists in the body positive movement started to combine fashion into their content, that's when we saw brands wake up and realize that fat women want to wear fashion too. We saw a huge expansion of the number of stores which offered plus sizes. And even though we are still lacking, it's come leaps and strides and I do feel we have been able to impact change."

With that said, Stephanie also explains how the most marginalized bodies, including many early architects of body positivity, now often find themselves excluded from the very movement they worked to build. "The body positivity movement as it is now has done a lot for mid-size women—but not so much for plus-sized women. This is no shade to the amazing models out there at the moment, but these small fat models who have exaggerated hourglass figures, big boobs, small waists, flatter stomachs, high cheekbones: they are the faces of body positivity. Somebody that looks like me doesn't necessarily fit into that. I'm not the biggest advocate of what body positivity has become now, because it is no longer a safe space for those who are the most oppressed to come together and talk about the stuff that really affects us."

The newest version of body positivity suggests that people should love their bodies *as long as they are healthy*, a vague standard that fails to contend with historic prejudices within the medical profession. "It's like, oh yeah, love yourself unless you aren't healthy, then you need to work on your health. Or love yourself unless you're *too* overweight. There are now a lot of conditions which pop up, which completely goes against the original ideas of the movement," explains Ally Duvall. Exclusion based on body size, shape, color, and ability continues, just in a different shiny guise.

Many have also found that the body positive conversation has become toxic and unwelcoming. Just consider the amount of criticism directed at Adele for losing weight and apparently betraying body positivity. "My body's been objectified my entire career," she said at the time. "I understand why some women especially were hurt. Visually I represented a lot of women. But I'm still the same person . . . I was body positive then, and I'm body positive now." Similarly, there was a lot of backlash from fans when Lizzo announced she was doing a juice cleanse. With so few women of size in the public eye, it's understandable that those who champion and embody different body shapes become icons and role models. But holding them to a new kind of standard yet again underlines that our worth is based solely on our body shape. Too big, too small, too tall, too short, too skinny, too curvaceous—any body standard is toxic, and no person should feel pressured to eat or move or be a certain way. No one wins in that game.

If I'm being honest, my initial reaction to both Lizzo and Adele was *nooooo!!* simply because I know the mindset that accompanies cleanses and dramatic body changes in my own life. But then I took a step back and reminded myself that everyone gets to choose how they interact with their own body. Losing weight does not mean you are anti–body love, just as gaining weight does not mean you are unhealthy. While I may not agree with everything a public figure chooses to promote, I must also recognize that 1) I don't know what's going on with that person, and 2) often people who believe they need to change to be happy are those I am trying to help, and judgment doesn't support my mission.

When it's just you and the mirror, the resounding reality is that sometimes you just don't feel that positive about your body. Yes, you can fight the voices in your head, argue with the unrealistic standards that have been set, disown the marketing messages you are fed on the daily, but wiping them from your memory is challenging at best. For some, toxic positivity can add a layer of guilt and shame—when we have those days that we don't feel positive about our body, it can feel like we failed. We begin pinching at our tummies or crying over a now-too-small pair of jeans, and suddenly we don't feel like the feminist, modern, hear-me-roar person who lives and breathes body positivity.

"I heard the sentiment of 'love your body,' and that felt to me like another standard that we couldn't achieve and I was letting myself down again," admits Alex Light. "Everyone else seemed to be loving their bodies and I was seeing all these Instagram posts every day telling me to love my body, so why didn't I? It made me see the beauty in other bodies that didn't fit the ideal. But I still couldn't apply that to my own body, and that is where I think the toxic positivity comes in."

While loving yourself in all your glory every day is an amazing goal, you should never feel like you've fallen short if you don't get there. You can have a bad body image day and still be a badass. If you do feel that way, or someone else makes you feel that way, that is the point at which body positivity becomes toxic. It is better to live in truth than to lie to yourself, no matter how hard that truth might be to accept.

A different track

So where does body neutrality fit into the equation? Neutrality could be described as the midpoint between body shame and toxic positivity—where the pendulum stops swinging. But I prefer to see it as existing on a totally different track, because unlike the two poles which are body-centered (bodily hate vs. bodily love; hate your stretch marks vs. love your stretch marks), neutrality takes the body out of the equation. No matter how we feel on any given day about our body—whether our pendulum is swinging toward deep shame or extreme positivity—the body neutral practice is to **acknowledge** the feelings we have, **explore** why those feelings may have shown up for us in the first place, and then **reconnect** with our self-worth.

I find examples can be really helpful when distinguishing body shame, body positivity, and body neutrality from each other, so here is a common scenario:

Body shame is walking past the mirror and talking negatively about yourself—it may sound like: *my stomach looks gross, I hate my legs, these stretch marks are ugly.*

Body positivity is countering those thoughts with positivity—think along the lines of: *my stomach is beautiful, I love every inch of my legs, stretch marks are my tiger stripes and they are great.*

Does countering body shame talk with body positive talk make you feel good? Do you believe it every single time? Does renaming your stretch marks something trendy make you love them? Sometimes, the answer is no. And sometimes the answer is yes! I know from experience that sometimes body positive talk really helps, and every so often you need to fluff yourself up so you can get yourself out of the house and on to the next thing. And yet, sometimes body positive talk can make you feel a little empty, as though you just lied to yourself.

Which brings us to the third option—neutrality. A body neutral response to negative thoughts may go something like this:

> *I'm really having a lot of negative feelings about my body.* (**Acknowledge** your feelings without judgment.)
>
> *I wonder why these thoughts are coming up so strongly today?* (**Explore** the hidden reasons—stress, lack of sleep, emotional distress, sickness, societal wiring, hormones, etc.)
>
> *I'm going to be extra gentle with myself during this time. My body is experiencing so much and yet it is still able to _____.* (**Reconnect** with yourself, and thank your body for what it does for you.)

These are the three practical steps we can take when we struggle to help mentally balance the ship: acknowledge, explore, reconnect.

Step 1:

Acknowledge your feelings

Tune in to the way you speak about your body and attempt to be a bystander to your thoughts:

Wow, I am having a lot of feelings about my legs today.

I'm listening to the things I'm saying about myself and I'm being really hard on myself right now.

The things that I'm saying I would never say to a friend.

The things I'm saying I would never say to my child.

These are nasty, hurtful things to think and speak.

Giving space to your thoughts can be eye-opening, which is why writing them down can reveal the reality of your relationship with your body in ways you maybe hadn't realized existed. Write down the thoughts you're not supposed to tell anybody. Stare at them, no matter how much you'd like to look away.

I always found the acknowledgment phase challenging because I didn't want to say many of those thoughts out loud. I didn't want to acknowledge that I was having a hard time. I wanted to have an easy time, I wanted to be strong and doing great and to love myself, no matter what. I wanted to believe I had achieved body positivity, job done, on to more fun things. But it's so important to tell yourself on the days you can't make it there, that it's okay to not be okay. I repeat, *it is okay to not be okay.* There's no shame in having a hard time—in the context of the world we live in, it's almost inevitable. Laying it all out and being really honest with yourself is the first step, because if you choose to suppress those thoughts and silence your true feelings, you can never get to the heart of what is really going on within.

The acknowledgment phase is, however, different from shame. Let's take the example of trying on clothes and finding you can't fasten the zip on one of your favorite dresses. Shame in that instance can throw you into a spiral. You can find yourself walking around your bedroom thinking, *I am disgusting,* and *I did this to my body,* and *I need to change all of this.* You can get caught in a mental frenzy of self-abusive language. That is very different from stopping to recognize and consider your feelings, which is more: *I just tried something on that didn't fit and now I'm really beating myself up about it.* It is one thing to be within the shame cycle and internally yelling at yourself. It's another to take a step back and acknowledge that you are yelling at yourself about your body. It is less heated, more dispassionate: *This is what my body shame sounds like today. This is what I'm saying to myself today. Wow, I'm really having a hard time with this.*

It's not that this first step makes you feel great, but it can help neutralize what's going on and help you detach a little. Acknowledgment is about pulling yourself out of the situation, standing up above yourself, looking down and seeing what's happening on the ground right now. Sometimes it helps me to view myself as different versions of myself. I'll think, *What age is feeling this right now? Which Bethany is showing up here? Am I acting as my teenage self or an earlier self?* Then I try to recruit another part of myself to speak compassionately to that side of me. Often, adult Bethany shows up to comfort young Bethany, and this is helpful because it reminds me that these feelings arise from former traumas or beliefs that I am now equipped to handle.

Maybe it's easier for you to think of it as a friend showing up to comfort you. What would they say, and what would you say back? The point of the acknowledgment phase is to allow space for you to really assess what's going on and hopefully take the first step to seeing it from a different perspective.

Step 2:

Explore where these feelings are coming from

There are two ways to do this. The first option is an in-depth exercise where you take the time to look at how your relationship to your body has changed over the years. I've left questions throughout this book in case you'd like to begin reflecting on some of your own thoughts as you read. I love the idea that this book is not just mine, but yours as well.

The other option is to perform an exercise in the moment. Ask yourself: *What else is really going on here? Am I extra stressed? Have I had an argument with my partner? Did*

I have to buy a bigger size in my jeans and that brought up something for me? Are my hormones influencing me strongly?

For example, say a relative made a comment about your body and now you are spiraling. You stepped away and acknowledged the feelings that you're having. Now you are exploring what is going on that is causing them: the obvious (Aunt Sue commented on your weight) and the less obvious (it's the holiday season, and you're not grounded in your normal routine). There will likely be many factors that you uncover in the explore phase, because it is rarely just one thing, so allow yourself to make a list. For example: holidays bring up feelings of loneliness; work has been extra challenging; I am staying in a home that isn't mine; I am experiencing a lack of control.

Recently, I was going through infertility treatments, and hormones were being pumped into my body daily while I was dealing with the fallout of medical procedures and failed pregnancy attempts. It was really hard to find acceptance in my body when I felt like it had betrayed me. When you're experiencing infertility, it's not just the inability to conceive, it's the complete lack of control you feel when it comes to your body. Nothing has ever made me feel so infuriated and so stuck. We'll dive into control more deeply later in this book, but we should note that feeling out of control is a major factor when it comes to body dysmorphia, eating disorders, disordered eating, and overall body shame. It's not a surprise that I struggled to ward off old patterns of thinking.

Whatever makes the list during your exploration phase, it is all valid. Some of the reasons that come up for you will just be unavoidable stuff that is going on in your life. Other times there are specific things you can eliminate from your life—standing on a scale, for example. I have no idea what I weigh, as I know for a fact that standing on a scale makes me spiral to a dark and addictive place that I don't care to go. After I realized this, I wrote an Instagram post about it, announcing that I wouldn't step on scales anymore—but while it was a public post, it wasn't really for anyone but myself. Voicing it helped hold me accountable, and I have not stood on a scale since. Even when I go to the doctor, I ask them not to weigh me, or if they need to weigh me I request a "blind weigh." Most doctors won't bat an eye; you'll simply stand on the scale backward and they'll write down the number confidentially. Maybe one day I'll feel above the scale, as though I have conquered its power, but I'm not there yet, and that's okay.

Another trigger for many people is trying on old clothes. Perhaps the seasons have changed and it's time to get your summer fits out. But through your exploration practice, you are now aware that this is something that could derail you. Think about what you can do to help make yourself feel safe and supported: ask your best friend over and give them a heads-up that you're going to need a cheerleader that day, or blast your favorite music, or turn on your favorite show. If it's available for you, it could be helpful to buy a few new items so you have clothing that fits and you are already excited about. If you know an item is not going to fit, don't try it on just to see how small it is: that item is a thing of your past, and your present self is your most important self. It may also be encouraging to think about what you are going to do with clothes that no longer fit. Can you donate them to help someone in need? Maybe sell them to make some extra cash? Or give them to someone you know and love—nothing makes me happier than seeing my nieces strutting around in my hand-me-downs! Whatever you do, try on old clothes when you are feeling good about yourself and your body. This is a good activity for a body-positive day.

You aren't going to be able to insulate yourself from these feelings in every instance, but by exploring your personal hot buttons, you will at least learn to recognize them. And then, once you have traveled some ways through these thoughts, the final stage is to take a step back and reconnect with yourself.

Step 3:

Reconnect with your self-worth through gratitude

A few weeks before writing the first draft of this chapter, I was having a bad body image moment. So, as I got in the shower, I started going through the three steps. I acknowledged the nasty things I was telling myself, and then I started to explore why I was saying them.

My exploration brought up a million reasons, but I pinpointed the main source as feelings of failure and shame surrounding a miscarriage I'd had months prior. After that, it was time to focus on reconnecting with myself, and summoning gratitude for all that my body can do. My body had battled infertility, become pregnant, lost the baby, gone through a D&C to remove the pregnancy tissue, bled, contracted, and screamed in pain—and still come out the other side. I'd had my first period post-miscarriage, and I was grateful for my bleed which signified life. I was grateful for my soft tummy and even my hormones bouncing in every direction. I was grateful for the break we took from trying as my body healed, and I was grateful that my body was healing. I was resilient, a warrior, and a human still living, breathing, and experiencing life. I may not have been at my fittest, my happiest, or my strongest, but I was still *me*.

The reconnecting step will look different for everyone, but turning our focus onto all that our body does for us, instead of the way it looks, can be transformative. In contrast to the body positive mindset, where you might be asked to write down something you love about your body—I love my smile, or my shoulders, or my neck—the body neutral practice doesn't involve looking at your body from an aesthetic point of view at all. The reconnection phase of body neutrality is centered on what your body can do for you—or has done for you. It's more action-oriented. The body is magical simply because it keeps us alive and breathing and perceiving the world and others around us.

For me, it's about reconnecting with that primal side and what my body does for me fundamentally. It allows me to have these thoughts, these joys, these moments. It's not *I really hate my legs today, but I love my boobs!* Or, *my arms are great, shame about my butt.* That's all just window dressing for the innumerable ways our bodies serve us every single day. Showing gratitude is beautiful here, because it also helps us connect to the present and be aware of all we have in this moment.

Activist and author of *See Me Rolling,* Lottie Jackson, explains how disability intersects with a body neutral practice. "When you are grappling with health issues there's sometimes a lot going on that constantly brings your focus back to the body. But if circumstances allow, it is possible to make your body neutral in the sense of mentally deprioritizing it and switching off for a while. For example, I have reminded myself that there is so much more to discover and enjoy beyond the physical constraints of your body. Whether it's using your imagination, being creative, connecting with people, or discovering new passions, the fleshly body is only one part of who we are."

After these three steps, there will inevitably be some kind of mental recalibration. Looking your feelings straight in the eye often takes the sting out of them. Yet moving through the three steps isn't going to make you think, *Yay! I feel great now! Sooo body neutral, off we go.* I explored these steps more days than not recently, and it was a few months of not feeling great and not feeling as body neutral as I might have hoped. But allowing myself the time and space I needed to feel those feelings and be in them helped me overcome them. It's not that the feelings disappear, but rather that you develop an emotional muscle memory that enables you to process and understand them.

Happiness comes from honest acceptance

My personal pendulum has swung all the way, hitting walls on both sides. Body shame? Been there. All the way there. Body positive? Been there too. Toxically positive. Does my pendulum now quietly rest at neutral all the time? Hell no. But am I breaking walls anymore? Thankfully, also no. I do want to be transparent about the fact that sometimes it's just *hard*, which can be difficult to confess. As the writer of this book and as an "expert" on movement and body politics, I often feel like I'm supposed to have it all figured out—and it feels strange to admit to you that I still struggle too. However, having body neutrality as a backbone for my thoughts—something I can always come back to—has helped me immeasurably, and I truly hope it can help you too.

At the end of the day, there is always something to strive for and there is always something to improve upon—that's the way our world is set up. But happiness doesn't come from self-harm or self-abuse or self-delusion. Happiness doesn't come from restriction and punishment, self-hatred and shame. Happiness doesn't come from shitting rainbows and pretending that we love ourselves every single day when actually we're struggling. Happiness comes from honest acceptance, something that body neutrality has the power to help you find.

CHAPTER 2

Body Bias

All bodies are created equal, but they are not treated equally

Now that we have established the principles of body neutrality, it's time to look at the world outside of our bodies. The reality is that, no matter how we feel within our skin, the way we look impacts how we are treated by others. Our relationship with our body doesn't exist in a vacuum. None of us are born with inherent beliefs about body shape, size, color—instead they develop through how we are treated, or see others being treated.

Over the course of my career, I have noticed how others are discriminated against in all areas of life. Fitness instructors of a bigger size who are not taken seriously, or clients in larger bodies who cannot get the care they need from their health providers. I've seen how a thin person can walk down the street eating an ice cream cone without an ounce of judgment from the people they pass, and a fat person cannot. Those living in larger bodies are subjected to negative discrimination in employment, education, healthcare, and even in relationships. And we have to wonder how much harm this constant judgment must do to the overall mental and physical health of a person. Mark my words: health is not about how someone looks, and the ways we gauge health in our communities need to be reconsidered.

We live in a society that has led so many of us to feel collectively bad about our bodies, and people of every shape and size have difficulties, struggles, and problems with body acceptance. If you have a body, you have an experience. We each encounter different experiences due to the privileges we may or may not have—and no matter what form your body takes, there is benefit in exploring how you can help yourself and others. The more we put people into boxes, the harder it can be to see one another for who we really are and let down our barriers. As well as addressing systemic issues that impact our relationships with our bodies and our self-esteem, I hope we can be more aware and compassionate toward others as we explore how bodies are treated differently based on their appearance. By reflecting on how the world has responded to us, we can hopefully better examine how we respond to others.

A note on body neutrality

One criticism that is sometimes directed at body neutrality is that it fails to address the fact that, while living in a world which remains steeped in bias, practicing body neutrality will be faced with external resistance. "As long as fatphobia exists, I could wake up every morning, feel neutral about my body and go about my day, but there are going to be people who will do their best to shame me," Stephanie Yeboah explains. "That could be having people calling me fat in the street, but it could also be going to the supermarket and having people look into my shopping basket, or having people stare at me in the gym, or going to a restaurant and seeing people take pictures of me eating. I'm always going to be reminded that my weight is the reason why I deserve to be treated with disdain or disgust. Whether that is on a dating app or in how fat people are portrayed in the media, I can't escape it."

For many people with disabilities, there can be both physical and practical barriers to setting the body aside. Lottie Jackson offers another perspective. "As someone with a physical disability, most of the barriers to acceptance of my body don't exist within me—they exist in the built surroundings, and other exclusionary conditions of modern life, that operate with a strict sense of how a body must move and behave. In this sense, I lack the control and agency to take full acceptance. Also, having a muscle weakness disability means that I have quite a unique and subjective experience of the physical world—I must always think about my body in ways that an able-bodied person may take for granted or see as instinctive. Simple actions like lifting a relatively heavy object require more effort and attention. Shifting the focus onto how a body functions, rather than how it looks, does imply some able-bodied privilege."

This book doesn't seek to invalidate these perspectives or suggest that body neutrality is a perfect "cure all ills" solution to systemic inequalities. It isn't. The aim of a body neutral practice isn't to forget about your body, but rather to find tools that help you respect your form while knowing it is not the most valuable thing about you. There may be some of you reading this book who find that the hurdles the world throws in your path are too high to be able to accept your body. That doesn't mean you have failed at being body neutral. Those feelings are valid and welcome here. With that said, there are people who live in marginalized bodies who find body neutrality to be a powerful practice that supports their journey toward healing their relationship with their body. I hope that there are aspects that you can take from body neutrality that might help you get closer to self-acceptance—even if they don't fully bridge the gap.

Ally Duvall credits body neutrality with helping her move from a deeply disordered relationship with her body into the acceptance she now feels. "Finding neutrality enabled me to let go of many of the things that I'd learned to attach to bodies. Exploring love for myself at a cellular level, a level that doesn't have anything to do with how I look in that moment, has been so rooted in the idea of neutrality, because it doesn't shift or change based on other factors. It doesn't care if I wore a different outfit, or if my pants are a little tighter in the way they hug my body. It's not this conditional way of being in the world: it just is."

One thread you will find me returning to in this book is that of curiosity and experimentation. Body neutrality may not be the single key that unlocks your own self-acceptance, because of the additional pressures your body experiences due to its shape, size, color, or ability. But it may offer a space for you to explore new techniques that could support you along the way. The environment you live in might be hostile, and yet there are ways you can protect yourself against some of the messages that come your way. A good starting point for accessing this shield is to look at the myriad ways that a body neutral practice can intersect with race, gender, size, and disability and help create a safer and more equitable space.

As Lottie says, "It is society that tells us our body is a measure of the quality of our existence. I guess realizing that is the first step toward reaching body neutrality—though I appreciate it's a lot easier said than done."

So, let's start with the landscape as it stands.

How the media marginalizes bodies

Our society accepts and even sanctions a huge amount of discriminatory behavior. Many of the organizations that define our opportunities for success and fulfilment operate with deep-rooted biases—from fatphobia to gender and racial inequity. "Bodies encounter remarkable bias," argues Chase Bannister, a licensed clinical social worker and president of the board of directors for the Eating Disorders Coalition for Research, Policy & Action. "We have bias against bodies of different sizes, shapes, colors, and appearances. A remarkable amount of body shaming and stigmatization happens all around us, which is often accepted as part of the backdrop of life rather than a particular hierarchy specific to this moment. Disenfranchisement bears its influence in potent ways when it comes to body weight, shape, size, and appearance: ways in which those walking through life in bodies which are accepted by their society can barely comprehend. But these messages have an impact on all of us, whether we acknowledge them or not."

If you aren't in a marginalized body, perhaps you've missed some of these messages. Perhaps you have wondered if the inclusion of larger body shapes in advertising and marketing promotes "obesity." Maybe you've felt defensive about being told you were wrong to encourage a friend who is proud of her weight loss. You were trying to make her feel good about herself, after all. Potentially, you've thought it's better that doctors are honest with those in larger bodies about the risks to their health. Quietly, you might acknowledge that you have little experience with non-binary or trans bodies, so you feel confused with how to refer to them or treat them respectfully. Many of the ways we have been taught to perceive bodies are based on insufficient research and assumptions, and it can be disorienting to unravel ideas that have been presented to us as fact. Many of us reading this are unlearning deep-rooted beliefs that have been passed down for generations—and that's hard! But it's part of this journey, and I encourage you to write down any feelings or questions that may come up as you read this chapter—and indeed the rest of this book. The hope is that it helps you reflect on and begin to change the way you speak about yourself and others.

A review of the past fifteen years of media found that, from television shows to books, newspapers to the internet, the media portrays people who live in larger bodies in a stigmatizing manner. "The media is the first port of call when it comes to how we identify and look at other people in the world," says Stephanie. "Growing up in the 1990s and 2000s, I always saw these evil characters that were fat or for some reason deemed ugly. All the goodies were slim and white and very attractive, and what that told me is that if I want to fall in love or be a hero in my story, I need to look like this specific type of person. Not every lead character in a romantic comedy needs to be white and slim—you can have a fat person as a love interest. You can have a disabled person as a love interest, or an Asian person as the love interest. We need to have TV shows and books and films that are more diverse with casting. If you have a platform in the online space, you also have a responsibility to change these messages."

Of course, media can also be a channel for positive change. Lottie describes using social media as "a vital means of being creative, staying connected, and seeking involvement in community." It is also the way that many of us engage with ideas beyond societal norms. "Social media has many faults, but finding a community online was the best thing that had ever happened to me," Stephanie agrees. "Because it taught me that normalizing fatness and bigger bodies is one of the key ways to bring home self-love. The body acceptance movement on social media was the place I found people who helped me love myself unapologetically. It showed me other plus-sized Black women—influencers and models who were a size 24 or 26 and who were living their lives fully and unapologetically. To normalize that on my social media feeds made me feel more at home with my body. I didn't see it as an anomaly or something weird and shameful anymore. It helped with my self-worth and that was something that I wanted to impress upon others as well. And I'm still flying the flag for it and trying to get my voice heard."

Health beyond size

A self-identified fat client once told me they had been experiencing knee pain. Every time they went to the doctor, they weren't provided with any treatment: the doctor just told them they needed to lose weight. After months of worsening pain, they finally saw a different doctor, who ordered an MRI and discovered they had a torn meniscus. I've thought about this a lot. Because I know for a fact that if I went to the doctor, I would be given an MRI for my knee without a second thought. We often hear about the causal relationship between increased body mass and negative health outcomes, but what is rarely mentioned is how consistently humans living at a higher body weight are misdiagnosed. It's unsurprising that many in larger bodies choose to avoid seeking medical advice entirely.

Nina Kossoff, an NYC-based strategist, consultant, and collaborator, speaks to that experience. "In high school I was captain of the swim team, and I was swimming for hours nearly every day of the week. I was also a vegetarian. That year at a routine checkup, my doctor told me that I was overweight and that I needed to work out more and eat more lean protein. They assumed I must be unhealthy with terrible exercise and eating habits without asking me about my lifestyle. The experience turned me off seeing doctors for a long while. I didn't get any say in what they wrote in my record. I was fat and so I needed to lose weight to be healthy. But how was I unhealthy? Was there something wrong with me?"

It doesn't matter if you're the picture of metabolic health with fantastic blood work, a solid sleep schedule, low alcohol intake, tons of stamina, low stress levels, and a great relationship with movement: we have been told that we can't be healthy without being thin. "A few days before a medical checkup, I was doing some DIY and knocked into a wooden table, so I had a bruise on my thigh which was slowly going away," recalls Stephanie. "At the checkup, the doctor saw the bruise and told me that one of the symptoms of super obesity was blood pooling—basically that I randomly get bruises because I'm fat. I explained to him that the bruise was a DIY injury, and it had nothing to do with a preexisting condition. I am told endlessly to lose weight even though there is nothing wrong with me, and it ranges from small things like the bruise to much bigger issues."

She continues: "A few years ago, I wanted to check my egg reserve because I've always wanted children. I went for a fertility test and the male gynecologist said that he thought my results were going to come back negative because I have so much fat around my hip section. He suggested I look at losing weight because obesity can decrease fertility, and that if I did want to have kids, I should lose about ten stone [140 pounds]. Needless to say, I was shitting myself for the next three weeks. It got to the point that I was crying and looking into diets again, which was something I hadn't done for years. And then the doctor calls me, sounding a little sheepish, to tell me that the tests came back perfect: my eggs were fine. I called him out on it and told him that he had made me feel terrible, and that for him to have assumed that I was infertile because of my weight was rooted in fatphobia. He simply said he had to tell me it may be a factor. But he didn't need to put that shame on me, especially before the results even came."

Yes, there can be negative health outcomes from living in a larger-sized body, just as there are from living in an undernourished and thin-sized body. There are also negative outcomes from many life choices and genetic predispositions which are not demonized. Light daily alcohol drinking (cancer, liver disease, heart disease, stroke), lack of sleep (dementia, heart disease, type 2 diabetes), even male pattern baldness (increased risk of heart disease and prostate cancer) can lead to negative health outcomes—and yet we're rarely shaming cocktail-bar goers, night owls, or bald dudes for being potentially unhealthy or dismissing their health concerns.

We live in the age of wellness, and health seems to have taken on a moral character. The result is those who are seen to be choosing their ill-health or potential ill-health are deemed immoral and bad people. What this fails to acknowledge is that attaining "health" isn't a possibility for some people, and many factors—including location, income, and socioeconomic status—can make it difficult or even impossible to access.

"I felt that doctors knew everything about health, so they must be right—I just needed to stop eating because I had to be healthy, or I must be a bad person," says Ally Duvall. "It's not only the big bad corporate diet media industry. It's leaders in our communities. It's the research that is being created. It's the focus on the obesity epidemic. All of these parts are continually building the message that fat people are bad and don't deserve care. When I was being treated for an eating disorder, my doctor didn't or couldn't look past my size. They never thought that I was someone who needed help with an eating disorder. Instead, they saw someone who needed help to lose weight."

The point is, "health" does not look one particular way, and our bodies are not business cards. When we assess people based solely on the way they appear outwardly, we overlook so many important factors and create a difficult environment for healing. Healthy or not, every single person deserves access to care. Each and every one of us deserves to be treated with respect and consideration—no matter what.

Setting boundaries to protect yourself

From preschool to the employment market, from dating sites to financial systems, the way we are treated is based on a web of value judgments. So how can we protect our mental well-being? I'm not going to pretend that I have the solution to the litany of biases every human

I Am More Than My Body

encounters and perpetuates—or that such a solution exists and can be explained in a few pages. But there is plenty within the body neutral mindset that can help us prepare ourselves to confront a biased world.

Step one is to acknowledge the impact these biases have on our self-perception and to interrogate them. "Over the past six to seven years, it's been dramatic to see how much systemic issues—whether it's race or religion or gender identity and sexuality—are coming into the therapy room," explains Dr. Pooja Lakshmin, a board-certified psychiatrist who founded the women's mental health community Gemma. "I only work with people that identify as women, and we are certainly under-standing that this isn't our fault. It isn't just anxiety or depression; we are living in a system that was not built for us—especially if you are a person of color—and we don't have any ways to navigate the world when we are burdened with this collective trauma. Our biggest tool to confront these issues is to create boundaries—true boundaries, not faux ones—to protect ourselves."

Let's address an example which came up time and time again in my interviews: going to the doctor and subsequently being told to lose weight. A person suffering from disordered eating might be guided by a professional therapist to body neutrality and be steered away from focusing on their body and weight as part of their recovery journey. They might finally begin to come to terms with their physical self, only to then be confronted by a doctor telling them to lose weight—not because they are displaying any particular ill-health, but simply because the scale says so. As a reminder, unless there is a medical necessity (for example, to determine the dosage of a medication), you have the right to refuse the scale.

It can be helpful to examine your personal triggers and create boundaries to protect yourself. Maybe this means having a conversation with your doctor about their practices before seeing them in person, or finding a network online to help you source practitioners who actively reject fatphobia. Or maybe it means attending appointments with a trusted friend. Setting boundaries is an active form of self-care, and a health booster in and of itself.

I loved this story Alex Light shared with me about a time when body-acceptance practice and boundary-setting helped her overcome a negative medical experience:

"I went to the doctor about my skin eczema, and he ended up telling me I needed to lose weight and I was so triggered by it. And then I was stunned that I felt so triggered because I have done all this work to improve my relationship with my body. What was cool to see is how quickly I was able to get over it. I felt sad and I sat with it, and I picked myself back up. I wish there was better advice, but practice is the only thing that has helped me. It does get easier and the armor does build up gradually."

Be compassionate to yourself and others

As for how to deal with the constant barrage of biased and often hurtful messages, Pooja suggests taking time to acknowledge how hard that task truly is. "Even when you intellectually know that you want to come from a more inclusive, compassionate stance, you have to start by recognizing up front what you are working through. For many of us, that is decades of talking to ourselves in a certain way based on how we have been treated. On top of that there are centuries of racism, sexism, ableism, and all of the -isms. Before you start to go interior, I think it is always important to preface these conversations with how difficult it is from the exterior. We have to be compassionate with ourselves about these truths."

Self-compassion is a wonderful practice that we will explore throughout this book. Lottie describes some of the ways that self-compassion has been a tool to reframe cultural scripts foisted upon her while growing up. "Self-compassion has helped me come to the realization that my disability and my body have shaped me in ways that are fundamentally positive," she explains. "I do not deny nor shy away from the fact that having a disability brings its frustrations and challenges. But I also know that it has given me a unique outlook on the world, which is something I can take pride in. Whether it's my problem-solving skills, uncovering beauty everywhere, extracting humor from a scenario, or expressing compassion and empathy, these facets of my identity have all arisen through navigating the world with a disability. To me, the knowledge that I have accrued these positive qualities is an act of self-compassion and internal validation."

Before we judge anyone or compare their struggles with our own, we have to understand how much of human experience is unquantifiable. We have never walked in their shoes. We have no idea about their genetic heredity, traumas, or mental health issues. We don't know what their parents said to them at the dinner table or how other kids treated them at school. We cannot scan their experience to see the influence of an abusive partner, or the jellyfish stings of a frenemy. While we seek compassion for ourselves, we should simultaneously hope to find compassion for others, no matter their appearance.

"We cannot create neutrality just for ourselves without creating full neutrality and full freedom for everyone," Ally explains. "It is not an accepting space or world until it accepts everyone. If you're simply body neutral toward yourself, you absolutely could have other biases that show up and that could be stigmatizing someone else. There are many fundamental issues with accessibility for people of my size. For example, when I go to a restaurant, I have to pre-research what it looks like outside. Do they have chairs that are accessible for me? There are many conversations around how we make this a space which is not only a space for me, but also for people who are more marginalized than me. People who are in a fatter body than me, who are a different race than me, and have different abilities to me. If you aren't engaging and challenging those issues then you aren't truly engaging with neutrality either."

When did you last consider how you speak to the people around you? If you have been speaking poorly to yourself and judging yourself harshly, how much of that is seeping out into your relationships with others? How do your comments about your own body impact the people around you who hear them? How far have you considered the experiences of other bodies in your day-to-day life? When you use travel systems or visit public venues, do you notice accessibility issues or challenge exclusionary policies? Have you ever thought about directing your custom toward spaces that prioritize inclusion? We cannot think about our own bodies differently without thinking about *every* body differently.

We live in a world where there is so much value placed on looking a certain way. It has been drilled into us that our appearance embodies so many facets of our identity.

How we look apparently signals our health, our virtue, our willpower, our success. To be neutral about our body is not only tough, but also an act of rebellion against a culture of 360-degree judgment. One of the most powerful and radical things we can do in this context is to begin to grapple with new messages and experiment with new practices. Playing with the notion that we don't have to love our bodies, that we don't even have to be happy with them—yet in the same breath acknowledging that we respect our bodies—smashes the system from the inside. Internalizing that this is the one body we have, and even if we're not always thrilled with how it looks, we can devote ourselves to caring for it, is game-changing.

This book alone is not going to fix systemic discrimination. But it can be the start of a journey to being more aware, more open to other people's experiences, and less fixed in the ways you see the world. Yes, it may always be a work in progress, but the narratives in your mind aren't immovable. In changing the way we treat ourselves, we can also change the way we treat others, so that we might begin to tackle this discrimination one step at a time.

CHAPTER 3

A Rebel with a Cause

All change starts from within

How our bodies are treated by society at large is one piece of the equation, but it's also important to consider how the external world can enter our mind and feel like an inner truth. We are a product of our society and our surroundings, which makes it tough to distinguish what we really want from what society tells us we should want. The repeated messages we hear from friends, family, media, professionals, and organizations can influence our self-worth, our identity, our deepest desires, and what we envision as being possible for ourselves. Addressing our internal dialogue is often the best place to start on the body neutral journey. It may feel overwhelming to think about changing the entire world to be a more welcoming and inclusive place, but we do have the power to shift the narrative going on between our ears. And the best part? Practicing body neutrality within ourselves can help influence those around us, and hopefully create a domino effect in our communities. All change starts from within.

Body neutrality in and of itself is an act of rebellion. Not being who the magazines, social media, entertainment industries, society—or anyone other than you—wants you to be has "rebel" written all over it. Much of this practice is about tuning out the noise and getting in touch with yourself. And this extends beyond weight and size, to body hair, wrinkles, gender expression, Botox, plastic surgery, and a million other things. What do *you* desire, when do *you* feel the happiest, what do *you* want and what truly serves *you?* Answering these questions is sometimes more difficult than we may think, but it can also be incredibly liberating.

This chapter in particular is going to focus on many of the standards set by the beauty industry, because they are preferences that we can experiment with and have agency over. The more we internalize that the only standards that matter are our own, the happier we can be with making decisions that truly support us.

Under the influence

I was born with a lot of hair. Like, a lot. One time, when I was a baby, someone at the grocery store mistook me for a furry animal (pretty sure my mom is still mad about this one). By nine years old I had dark, thick hair all over my legs, arms, and stomach. One evening, my brother and I were coming back from his basketball practice and his coach gave us a ride. I guess I was sitting on my brother's lap in the front seat (it was the nineties), and the coach looked down at our legs and said to my brother, "Man, your sister has hairier legs than you do!" The comment was supposed to be a dig at my brother—to say, *boy, you're not man enough, you barely grow hair on your legs*, but I felt it directed at me. Boys were supposed to have lots of hair, and girls were not. I still remember how mortified I was. That night I begged my mom to let me shave, and she did because she also felt embarrassed for me. I became the first child to shave in my class.

When I was around eighteen, laser hair removal hit the market and I was instantly hooked—to the point that it was my graduation present. Over the next seven years, my arms, underarms, stomach, legs, bikini area, and nipples would all undergo countless rounds of laser hair removal. But over time, something changed. I found that my perception of armpit hair started to shift in tandem with my coming out and exploring gender (even though I no longer believe body hair has anything to do with how "masculine" or "feminine" we are). I started to think it looked cute and, although I'm pretty sure it was because I saw Miley Cyrus sporting hairy armpits, clearly something was changing in popular culture too. In fact, in 2020 Mintel reported that one in four women under the age of twenty-five no longer shaves their armpits, in comparison to one in twenty back in 2013. I grew out my pit hairs and never looked back.

This dramatic shift was proof that I had never actually hated the way armpit hair looked: I had simply never seen it as an option for female-bodied people. Cyrus Veyssi, a non-binary Persian content creator and creative strategist, has this to say on the topic of body hair: "I grew up around many Americans and white people, but I also grew up around Persians and Persian women. Persian women in general have a lot of hair and still identify as highly femme. But I also have my Western cousins—they were made fun of for their hair in school and now wax every part of their body. I never coded body hair as being masculine or feminine and that's a reflection of my specific culture."

Much of what we deem as "acceptable appearance" is based on the culture we grew up in, the people we surround ourselves with, and the media we consume. Cultural differences in beauty standards play out on all levels: among age groups, organizations, and even from city to city. I lived in Texas for a few years, and learned that big hair never goes out of style there. As Dolly Parton said, "The higher the hair, the closer to God!" Trends come and go—perhaps you once loved the way you look with barely there eyebrows, then one day you find yourself drawing them on thicker, before breaking out your tweezers again a decade later. The point is, one is not inherently ugly and one is not inherently beautiful—it's all subjective, and it's okay to fluctuate with the times. We'll likely always be influenced by the environment we live in, the media we consume, and the trends we see around us, but on the other hand that doesn't mean we have to change things about ourselves that we love, or hate parts of ourselves if they're not in vogue. We are allowed to find beauty in the things that may not currently be deemed as "beautiful" by our cultural standards or media feeds.

To reflect on how your current view of beauty has been shaped throughout the years, here are some questions to consider as you read through this chapter:

What did beauty mean to you when you were young? Who were your beauty icons then, and who are they now? How are they different or similar?

When do you first remember feeling strongly about a physical attribute, beautiful or not?

How did the environment you grew up in influence the way you perceived beauty? Does it still influence you?

How has your gender influenced your beauty standards?

Have you ever wished to explore a beauty standard outside of what is deemed acceptable for your gender?

Seeing beauty in a new light

One of my dad's favorite stories to tell about me was from when I was about four years old. We were taking a walk together and we passed by a house that had been destroyed in a fire. Barely standing, singed and sooty, it stopped me in my tracks. "Daddy, isn't that house beautiful?" I asked him in amazement. At this part of telling the story he would always laugh loudly and say, "Oh, to see the world through the eyes of a child!"

I think about that often, and wonder how it would be if we could see the world through the eyes of someone who has not yet been impacted by external ideas of what is or is not beautiful. We know that society goes through a series of trends and turnovers that influence how we dress and look, but have you ever found your own perception of yourself dramatically shifting? I remember a time when I would never leave the house without mascara: I thought I looked ugly without it. Then one week I had an eye infection and couldn't wear mascara for a week. The first few days I didn't want to look at myself in the mirror, and then around day four, I saw myself in a new light. Suddenly my bare eyes looked beautiful to me. From that day on, I felt comfortable deciding whether or not I wanted to paint my lashes. It was no longer an obligation; it was a choice.

Cyrus opened up to me with a similar story of the expectations that they felt once they defined themselves in a new way. "Beauty has been extremely validating for me. At times I have tried to conceal parts of myself with makeup, and it has been gender-affirming for me to do so. But my relationship with beauty has changed over time and I'm far more relaxed about it," they say. "I used to feel if I was leaving the house, I *had* to affirm my gender and I *needed* to wear makeup no matter what. There are still times when I do feel pressure to have my full face on—like when I go to events with brands that I am working with. When you're not a cisgendered woman in this industry you are definitely expected to turn up 100 percent done. Don't get me wrong, going to CVS with the $20 I got from my allowance to experiment with makeup brought me out of some dark places. But sometimes I'm exhausted by the performance of it.

We can celebrate positive changes in the beauty industry while acknowledging the fact that it is stuck. Deconstruction of beauty norms is incredibly difficult, but whether it is helped by brands sticking a trans or non-binary person in there, though only if they 'look' trans or non-binary, is up for debate."

There are many ways to get closer to yourself. Whether it's massaging a patch of stretch marks or lovingly combing your gray hair or playing with that belly roll, touching your body in gentle and safe ways can be an excellent tool in reconnecting with your physical self. Experimenting can also be powerful: as Cyrus and I both experienced, trying different looks and aesthetics can be a fun way to figure out your unique preferences. Just be sure you are in a safe and nonjudgmental space when you are trying out new things. One of my favorite times to experiment is when I'm on vacation, because I'm removed from my everyday environment.

When I spoke to Stephanie Yeboah, she talked about how one of the main joys of living on her own has been to be able to spend time naked, and described it as a great way to reconnect with her body. "Walk around your house naked. Completely. All the time. For a day, an evening a week," she suggests. "As soon as I lived alone, I started doing it, and so quickly my body became just a thing. I stopped focusing on whether my boobs were saggy or how my stomach looked and I normalized my naked body for myself. That was such a great tool to help me see my body for what it is and not this thing that needs to be fixed. Spending time naked and looking at yourself how you are meant to be is so intimate and very powerful."

While often difficult, it is incredibly empowering to own your body as it is outside of what may be the current trend. Beauty really is in the eye of the beholder, which means that the standard of beauty is different for everyone. Often it's not our body that needs to change, it's our mindset.

The shame-guilt conundrum

With all this said, experimenting and exploring isn't always easy, and you might find that other people will have a lot to say about it. As the saying goes, "Damned if you do, damned if you don't." Often it may feel as though there is no winning: we feel ashamed for spending too much time beautifying ourselves, or ashamed that we don't carve out more "me" time. This is because society is mostly set up to be a lose-lose situation. I call this the shame-guilt conundrum. You can bet that no matter what your position, someone out there will tell you you're wrong. So how do we figure out what we really want without judging ourselves based on what we've been taught? How do we become curious about what makes us feel the most comfortable within ourselves?

After coming to terms with my armpits, I started feeling rebellious and decided to grow out my leg hair too. I was under the impression that, much like my armpit hair, if I grew accustomed to it, I'd soon grow to love it. Spoiler alert: I was wrong. I gave it two years: I grew it out and watched the hair turn long and dark and soft. I exposed it on red carpets, wore it to the beach, I dyed it a bright color a few times, and one summer I even glued multicolored gems to it (I have to be honest, that was pretty cute).

Even though I pretended to like the way my leg hair looked, deep down, I knew I didn't. Sure, I liked not spending time shaving. Yes, I liked saving money on razor blades. I definitely liked that it was a big middle finger to traditional gender roles, but even though I kept the hair for two years, I can't say I ever fell in love with it. Here I was doing something that went against what my society deemed acceptable because *I make my own choices and all else be damned!*—and yet I didn't actually like the choice I was making. When I was shaving every day, I felt frustrated that I was conforming to outdated beauty standards. And when I wanted smooth legs again, I felt frustrated for not adhering to my "progressive values." Both of these opposing beliefs left me with feelings of guilt—but, whether our choices are deemed radical or not, we should never feel guilty for making decisions that are right for us.

I loved hearing Cyrus's take on body hair. "Deciding to keep my facial hair has been an act of self-assertion. Because even though the non-binary identity is still in its nascence for the mainstream, there are already social standards for what a non-binary person should look like. But now, I have internalized the truth that wearing makeup does not make me non-binary and I can be non-binary with a beard. I feel so passionately that we need to de-gender external appearance. Sometimes I used to look in the mirror and think, *I need to throw on hoop earrings to offset this hair,* because I didn't look gender-fluid enough. Now I think, *enough for whom?"*

I really do believe one of the most radical and rebellious things you can do is to be neutral about your body. So often our bodies act as a battleground in a war of ideas, weaponized and politicized on all sides. How would it feel to let go of the weight of that burden, and allow your body to just *be*? To allow your aesthetic choices to be just that—simple choices—rather than having them be a flag about your beliefs on unrelated matters? To approach things like body hair and makeup without judgment, toward yourself or others? To forget what society thinks—and by that I mean what *all* of society thinks, from the most conservative to the most progressive. I want you to ask yourself: what makes the most sense for *your* life?

Neutrality for the win

Here's the cool thing about my leg hair journey: I no longer care about it like I used to. Yes, I prefer my legs to be hairless when I'm wearing a minidress, but I don't shave every day like I used to. In fact, I'm less bothered by hair generally. These days I let my hair grow freely, and when something big is coming up and I know my legs will be on display, I'll wax them myself in my bathroom. I don't mind wearing shorts with stubble, I don't panic-shave when my calves aren't covered, my leg hair no longer feels dirty or shameful, but nor does it feel proud or rebellious. I feel neutral about it: some days hair is there, and some days hair isn't, and I get to decide. As trivial as it may seem, it's an incredibly freeing feeling. I no longer *have* to remove my hair, I *get* to remove my hair—on my timeline, on my terms, in my way.

This is why getting closer to a neutral place is so rewarding; it releases space in our brain, allowing us to focus less on the physical stuff and more on the emotional, spiritual, mental stuff: the stuff that will better us as humans and enrich our lives. When exploring neutrality, it can be helpful to safely perform experiments on yourself. Maybe you don't grow out your leg hair for two years; maybe you grow it out for a month. Maybe you don't start by throwing out the scale at home; maybe you hide it for the summer. It can be liberating to break your own beauty standards, and notice what that does or doesn't do for you.

One year I took a very off-the-grid "vacation" to do some soul-searching. I stayed for a week deep in the jungle, in a place that could only be accessed by foot. There was no electricity, no running water, no cell service, and no mirrors. While I had planned to use my hand mirror or phone to look at myself each morning, upon arrival I got the urge to see if I could go the week without seeing my face. I was astounded by what a powerful experience that was. By day three I felt detached from my appearance, and I noticed the way that changed how I interacted with new people. I felt more myself, less conscious and more free. With my looks off my mind, I focused on making connections.

I'm not asking you to trek to the jungle or throw out your phone, of course, but if you find yourself constantly worrying about how you look or spending time in front of the mirror bashing yourself, what would it feel like to cover the mirrors in your home for a week? What would it feel like to limit the time spent staring at your reflection?

Give this experiment a try!

Step 1: What is one thing about your appearance that you feel self-conscious about? This could be anything from your hair length, to wearing makeup, to showing your legs. *I'm going to do this with you using my mirror example from above.*

Step 2: What would the opposite extreme of where you currently are look like? How does the thought of that make you feel? *This would be like imagining never having access to a mirror.*

Step 3: What would the midpoint between these two extremes look like for you? How does that make you feel? *That may be like only looking in the mirror once a month.*

Step 4: Keep going until you get to a change that feels manageable. Where is that point for you? *For me, that was not looking in a mirror for a week.*

Step 5: Now think about a time and a place where it would feel safe for you to try putting that into practice. *For me, it was only when I was in the jungle away from social media and work that I felt comfortable putting the mirrors away.*

Create an environment that feels protective and then try it out! You might be surprised at what you discover.

Connecting with your intentions

There are many reasons someone might choose to change their physical appearance—from minor changes like dyeing their hair to major ones like plastic surgery. It isn't up to us to judge their decisions. I know many people who have an issue with getting Botox: any type of injectable is off-limits and they believe anyone who gets it must not love themselves. To put it plainly, I think this is bullshit. I wholeheartedly believe that you can get Botox or plastic surgery and still love the hell out of yourself. I also don't think it's helpful to make up arbitrary rules and hard lines that might make people feel guilty. If I were to make you feel bad about the Botox you just got, would you want to lean in closer to my body neutral message, or would you prefer to go out and find friends who like Botox just as much as you? Probably the latter!

Have I seen people use plastic surgery as a way to try to bandage the deep shame they feel about themselves? Absolutely. Have I seen people who have gotten plastic surgery as a way to better themselves and feel more comfortable in their own skin? Absolutely. What we can do for ourselves is examine the intention behind our desire for change, and our expectation of the outcome.

I've loved talking with my friend Nina Kossoff about their top surgery. "I identify as non-binary and I've been lucky to have had an easy relationship with my gender in my body. This is by far not the experience of many trans or non-binary people, but I've always been quite matter-of-fact about how I feel in my gender," they say. "Making the decision to get top surgery wasn't that complicated. For me having a chest of any kind was a nuisance. I hated running while wearing two sports bras. That wasn't the entirety of it all—I wanted to connect to my body in other ways too—but I wasn't hyper-fixating on what didn't feel right. After I had the surgery, I felt like, *Oh lovely. I didn't like this part of me, I fixed that, and now I'll go on with the rest of my life.*"

I relate to how neutral Nina's approach is. Making any kind of change to your body is simply no one else's business. "If we are looking at bodies as a neutral thing, who cares if you change it?" they ask. "If someone is telling you not to change anything about your body and to love yourself exactly as you are, this is where positivity can become toxic. My gut reaction is, why do you care if it makes me feel more comfortable in my body? There are gender-affirming reasons for why people might adjust their bodies, and that's not just a trans and non-binary issue. People of all genders elect to do body modification surgeries to affirm their gender. They might get filler, or liposuction, or a nose job. The argument that your body is your home and therefore you shouldn't feel the need to change it can be flipped: if it is simply an outer shell, who cares if I change it? My surgery was like choosing to wear a lovely soft T-shirt instead of a terrible, scratchy one. I feel more comfortable, that's it. If there was something which would feel better for you day-to-day, then why not do it?"

A note I received recently from Lindsay Young Champion, one of my followers, is a great illustration of why and how body modifications aren't a black-and-white decision:

> Oh preacher of body neutrality, I'm struggling. 2+ weeks ago I had a breast reduction. Something I've wanted for over a decade. I was a 38H and it was affecting my life. I couldn't wear seat belts properly. I couldn't find bras that didn't make me bleed. My breasts hung down past my belly button. Post surgery, I love them. BUT how do I reconcile "respecting my body" when I surgically changed it? If I respected my body for exactly how she showed up for me pre-surgery, then why did I permanently alter her? I'm happy with my body now, but was it right for me to be unhappy with it before? Am I only happy because it's smaller?

This message broke my heart. I share the message of body neutrality, but I never want that to come across like we should feel guilty or ashamed for making active choices about our body that serve us. And that includes body modification. Altering our bodies is not inherently "wrong," just like dyeing our hair a different color is not a betrayal of our natural selves. More than examining the choices we make, we should examine the intention with which we make them.

It may be tempting to believe that having a smaller nose, a bigger butt, or fewer wrinkles is going to make you feel brand new. Yet unless we examine our intentions and expectations, very little that we do to our outsides has the power to change our emotional well-being in the long term. It's also helpful to be honest about the pressures which might have led you to make the decision in the first place. Especially when it comes to making permanent changes that may come with risk factors, it's worthwhile to be honest with yourself about why you are getting a procedure done. If it's for someone else, or because you think it will make you more popular or attractive or acceptable to another person, it may not be coming from a neutral place.

If you are considering surgery or any body modifications, connecting with your intentions and expectations can be a useful step. Here are some questions that might help guide you in your decision-making:

Is there a functional reason behind this modification? Is your main aim to make your life more comfortable (either physically or psychologically) or practical?

When you think about NOT getting it done, how do you feel? Does it feel shameful to remain in the body that you have? If so, try moving through the body neutral steps (acknowledge, explore, reconnect) and see what doing that brings up for you.

What are you hoping to get out of this body modification? What is your ultimate aim or goal? How do you think things will be different in your life beyond the changes that you're making?

Ultimately, what I hope this chapter has proved to you is that there is often value to be gained by experimenting and getting curious with yourself and your body. Sometimes the things that feel the most comfortable are the things that we have grown up seeing and which feel the most familiar. But that doesn't make them right for us, and it certainly doesn't mean that they will continue to serve us in the long term. What could you potentially gain if you explored outside the box and questioned a few of the beauty norms that you hold to be true? Remember, you don't have to stay there if it doesn't feel good—but the journey of experimenting might just change your mindset along the way.

CHAPTER 4

Childhood Stories

The smallest things can have the biggest impact

I was born and raised in a little pass-through town in Missouri called Festus. Festus is a typical small American town and, as in most places, food is what brought my family together. Dinners were made at home—or at Grandma and Paw Paw's house, where we'd gather around the table and eat his famous ribs and her famous pies. When we could afford it, we'd go out to dinner after church on Sunday. And like all good Midwesterners, we had meat and potatoes at every meal. Unfortunately for me, I'm one of the few people who positively *hates* potatoes. The texture has made me gag ever since I was a kid, and to this day I can't stand them. But given I was raised as part of the "clean your plate" generation, I was forced to eat potatoes at basically every meal. Each time, I would cry into my potato-filled plate, take an unwilling bite, and start gagging. And each meal I got in trouble for being "too dramatic" (to be fair, I *was* generally pretty dramatic—but this was the one time I wasn't performing), and was made to sit at the table until I finished supper. Often a lonesome hour would pass until my dad would come along, hungry once again, and eat them for me.

Consequently I became the family's "picky eater." I was labeled a difficult child who had problematic eating habits, rather than an opinionated child who simply didn't like some foods. "Parents often forget that every person, and that includes kids, has their own unique taste buds," says Megan McNamee, a registered dietitian specializing in maternal and child nutrition and eating disorders, and co-owner of Feeding Littles, a platform that offers advice to parents. "I think parents assume that if they like this food and this food tastes fine to them, then their kids should eat it too. But they don't know what kids are experiencing in their bodies, or what it tastes like to them. There are people who don't like biting into a blueberry because they don't like the squish feeling. At least 4 percent of the population has a gene that makes cilantro taste like soap. Some of us are super-tasters when it comes to bitter foods, so kale or broccoli truly taste disgusting. It's not obstinance—children's preferences are valid."

In fact, as Megan explains, parental pressure to eat can be incredibly self-defeating. Studies have shown that pressure to clear the plate is associated with patterns of both under- and overeating; that rewarding fullness with more food ("you have to finish your meal to get a dessert") reinforces poor eating habits; and that calling your child a problem or picky eater can further perpetuate their fussiness with eating.

The body talk that surrounds us as children has a huge impact on how we view our bodies as adults. "So many of my clients' first exposure to dieting was in the home," says Megan. Diet talk pervaded my family and seeped into my upbringing, as it does with so many. It was subtle—we didn't do a lot of restricting or calorie-counting—yet it was always present: body-bashing at the pool, labeling desserts as "bad," or seeing people of size as unfortunate. Sure, my picky eating was an annoyance at the dinner table, but it was also subtly envied by the adults because I had "self-control" and was a small size. Everyone loved me because I was tiny and cute: I was always placed at the top of the cheerleading pyramid, my brother's girlfriends made me up as though I were a doll, and any compliment I received focused on how little I was. I remember fearing getting bigger—even just growing at all—because who would pay attention to me then? Who would I *be*? Even before I was a fully fledged teenager, I had concluded that being small was my worth in this world, and gaining weight or being anything other than tiny was not acceptable.

Let's get something straight: I don't want this to come across as "Oh, poor baby me, I was soooo slim and little, feel sorry for me!" That's not the sentiment here. What I hope this story conveys is that the comments we make about children's bodies have lasting effects. Kids are more than their bodies (we all are!), and when we obsess about their size—big or small—we teach them that this is where their identity lies. We forget about their interests, their dreams, and their goals, and we hinder development by placing them in a box. They become *the tiny girl who is a dancer*, or *the fat kid who is funny*, or *the strong boy who plays sports*.

When I spoke to Johanna Kandel, founder of the National Alliance for Eating Disorders, she told me the poignant story of how her eating disorder began.

"At the age of three I was walking pigeon-toed, so my parents put me into ballet. Much to their dismay, I fell in love with ballet, and I ended up going to a special performing arts middle school and high school. When I was eleven, the artistic director of the professional company told us there was going to be a big audition and they needed us all to lose weight beforehand. I remember getting into the car that night with my mom and saying, 'I'm going on a healthy food diet and will be eating more fruits and vegetables.' Of course, if your child says they want to eat healthily, you're going to be supportive. But over time, I became more and more restrictive and, at a certain point, this tipped over into a ten-year eating disorder, which threatened my life both through suicide attempts and cardiac arrest. That one comment at such an incredibly young age set the wheels in motion for me." Johanna's story is a striking example of how the smallest things can have the biggest impact.

Here are five neutral ways to interact with kids that don't place their worth on their identity, ability, or appearance:

What are you playing with? Can you show me how it works?

Tell me about your friends!

Which would you rather have: wings to make you fly or shoes that make you run super fast?

I enjoyed spending time with you today!

What's something that always makes you laugh?

Break the cycle

I remember the first time I ever attended a weight loss meeting with my mom. I was around twelve, my dad had passed away a few years before, and she was getting remarried, which meant every wedding magazine was telling her she needed to be thinner. The weight loss meetings were through our church, a bible-study-slash-restrictive-food program. I can't remember why I was there—I was still a small-framed child—but I remember the class leader taking out a silicone model of what fat looked like, and it was this hideous, gross thing that made me physically nauseous. I learned then that fat was something to be feared, and from that day on I would mentally recall that silicone form as a way to curb my appetite and stop me from wanting to eat "bad food."

I need to caveat this story by expressing that I don't place any blame on my mother—not for her diets, not for taking me to these meetings, and not for any of the issues I would have later on in life. Like many parents, she did everything she could to raise me in the best way she knew how. "Many women have told me that what they find the most triggering are those comments from people that are close to them, like friends and family—often mums, grandmas, and aunties. And that is so difficult," Alex Light explains. "But I think we need to understand that they are also a product of their environments. Many of them spent their entire lives being faced with the idea that they needed to be thin. I think if you can realize that the issue lies with them and employ compassion, then I hope you will be in a much better place to have those comments bounce off you rather than internalizing them. But that is so tough and it's not an overnight thing. It takes practice."

Everything my mom did was out of love and with good intent. Sure, maybe in hindsight there are things she would want to change, but what parent wouldn't? Parents are continually learning and improving on their methods for raising their children. Mom, I love you and I'm grateful for every single one of our experiences together. Parenting is hard enough already without the need to start pointing fingers, and for any parent reading this, you should take a moment to pat yourself on the back and kiss your shoulders for simply showing up to read these pages. You are working to break the cycle passed down from generations before, and that is a beautiful thing.

Being aware of our own relationship with food is the first step that we—as parents, caregivers, or mentors—need to take if we want to break the cycle for younger generations. "Developing an awareness around this can be really tough, and there is a lot of guilt that can come up when we open our eyes to the non-dieting approach," Megan points out. "You might think, *Oh my gosh it's too late, I messed my kids up.* But you can always talk to them and say, for example, 'I know you've seen me weighing my food, but I've realized that's not good for me and that's not how I want to approach food anymore.' Or, 'I'd like to listen to myself and my own body now and eat the foods that feel good to me, and for you to do so too.' Kids are so adaptable, and it's not the end if you haven't always been modeling the most positive approach to food. Nobody knows it all."

I hope that as we work through this chapter, acknowledging and exploring the many different ways that children form beliefs around food, you will have the chance to reflect on the food stories you were raised on as well, and consider how they may still be influencing you.

Here are some questions to get you going:

What did mealtime look like for you as a kid? Did you eat together or alone? Did you enjoy the food you were served?

What did positive mealtimes look like? What did negative mealtimes look like?

How was your body spoken about when you were young? How have those comments impacted how you see yourself today?

What foods, if any, did you internalize as being "bad"? What foods did you internalize as "good"? How do you see these foods today?

What kind of relationship did members of your family (including generations past) have with their bodies?

Stepping outside the home

Even if we, as adults, are completely neutral in the way that we talk about bodies around the children in our lives, the difficult reality is that we cannot shield them from the kind of body talk that happens outside the home. "I have a nine-year-old whose friends are already talking about dieting. And I literally feel physically sick talking about it because it can happen so young. The moral is that the messages from the outside world come through earlier and a lot stronger than we think," says Megan.

School is where many of us first see how many different shapes and sizes humans come in. If kids see that smaller-sized bodies are praised in gym class or tryouts, they will hold the belief that smaller-sized bodies are better. If they are told that the way they move is incorrect or not valuable, it is likely they will develop a negative relationship with movement. Nearly everyone I spoke to for this book had a memory from their early school days that impacted the way they related to their body for years—and sometimes decades—after that.

"My entire relationship with movement was destroyed as a child because I had horrible gym teachers. We were lined up and forced to do as many pull-ups as we could to compare our abilities. The answer was zero for me, and the experience made me feel like total shit," Nina Kossoff recounts. "By seventh grade, I had been swimming for a long time, and I continued to be a competitive swimmer for many years after. But because of the way my body looked, my gym teacher would call me out during class and say, 'When you swim six days a week, why can't you run a mile?' There was a total lack of understanding that running was an entirely different type of movement, and it left me with the message that it wouldn't matter what I did, because I couldn't move in the way that counted."

But it's not just school. Doctors' offices are another place where many can experience body shame early on. "So much of my own experience came through a doctor telling me to lose weight," recalls Ally Duvall. "I would never have even questioned that, because that is a person who is in a job with power, they are leaders in our community. So, if they say I need to go on a restrictive diet at eleven, before I've even gone through puberty, I sign up to Weight Watchers without questioning it. That experience kicked off my eating disorder and years of total misery."

Over the past decade, our 24/7 "always on" digital culture has transformed our interactions with all kinds of cultural messages, and this is especially true for children and young people. Globally, one in three internet users is under eighteen, and their chances of contact with harmful and disturbing content increase the more time they spend online. "I'm not surprised by the volume of what we have called pro-ana [pro-anorexia] or pro-mia [pro-bulimia] content online," says Chase Bannister. "When you think how many are suffering, to suggest there shouldn't be such sites is tantamount to saying there shouldn't be mental illness. I'm always very careful to be thoughtful about using the language of 'good' or 'bad' in these contexts. A pro-eating-disorder site is where we might find the folks that we would hope to care for. As problematic as this content can be in potentially catalyzing more damaging behaviors, let's be cautious not to shame the creators for their mental illness."

What has surprised Chase is how social media companies have monetized the high level of engagement such content generates. "We now know that social media companies are making a lot of money through advertising connected to these [pro-ana, pro-mia] spaces. Instead of seeking to limit its circulation, they are profiting from its popularity amongst children, and that's just not okay."

This can seem terrifying to anyone hoping to protect young people, but it's not all doom and gloom. While we cannot—and nor should we want to—police children's every move, we *can* set them up with the foundations of neutral thinking when it comes to their relationship to their body and to food. These values may not prove unshakable, and it will be ongoing work. But understanding that there are different ways to perceive bodies and learning that food doesn't have to be laden with moral judgment can lead to higher psychological well-being and a lower incidence of disordered eating behaviors.

"We can only control what is said and done in our home. And that is more impactful than what they are going to see in the outside world," says Megan McNamee. We have the power to change the story, for ourselves and for future generations.

Looking to the future

I think about future generations and how all of us, whether we are parents or not, have a responsibility to make the world a better place for them. (A note on language: in this next part, when I write about "girls" and "boys," I'm coming at it from the point of view of biological sex assigned at birth, and not gender identity—which one may choose to explore.) I've been blessed with thirteen niblings (nieces and nephews) in my family: ten girls and three boys so far. When I was a child I was surrounded by boys—there hadn't been any girls born into the Meyers family for several generations, until my cousin and I came along. So when my brothers started having kids and we suddenly had a plethora of girls in our family, I was over the moon.

A couple of years ago, I had my birth chart read (I highly recommend doing this if you're a curious, star-loving person like myself). My chart indicated that my purpose on this earth is to break a generational cycle of thinking for the women in my family, and that really stuck with me. When I started my own fitness platform, the be.come project, my nieces were always in the back of my mind: Would I want them to do this workout? Would I want them to hear the way I speak about my body? As I write this book, I think about all of the women and girls in my family. Would I want them to read these words? Could the practices in these pages help support their own body acceptance? How does our body neutral journey affect the generations of littles following in our footsteps?

The best way to model a body neutral approach for young people is simply to practice body neutrality in our own lives. "We recently rolled out a parents' body image program that we do for families at Equip," says Ally Duvall. "So parents can look at their own relationship with their bodies, and work on that as they support their child in treatment. That is vital, because if a child works on their own body image but goes back into an environment that doesn't support that, it's going to be really tough for them."

Does this mean we all need to master neutrality, positivity, or acceptance in every single situation before interacting with kids? Of course not! That's an impossible standard, and kids don't need us to be perfect; they need us to show them how to grow, change, and learn. They need us to show them that sometimes body neutrality is really hard, and that's okay. In Megan's words: "Even if we are still working on our own stuff, we can honor body neutrality for them."

In practice, this means being mindful of the language we use around young people to describe bodies, diets, and health. "My biggest piece of advice," says Megan, "is, if you can't say anything nice about your body in the mirror in front of your child, just don't say anything at all. Or at least do your very best to keep your language body neutral when you're talking about yourself in front of a child."

To get you started, here are some body neutral ways to talk about clothing next time you're getting dressed or going shopping with a young person. A good tip is to focus on the *function* of your clothes.

> This outfit keeps me warm.
>
> I feel so comfortable in this dress.
>
> These jeans make my body feel supported.
>
> This doesn't fit me anymore so I'm going to wear something else.
>
> I'm going to try this on in a bigger size so my body can move more freely.

What this doesn't mean is shutting down all body conversations or avoiding talking about bodies altogether. I often think about a story that Ally shared with me when we spoke. "I was at the pool this weekend, and a child made a comment about my body. It's a developmentally appropriate skill for children to describe what they are observing, but it might be challenging for parents to hear their kid declare, 'Oh my gosh that person is big! Their belly is gigantic.' Parents will try to shut the conversation down, and that can shift a child's understanding of cultural acceptance. It makes being fat something taboo. Going back to my pool trip this weekend, I responded by saying, 'I know! I have a big belly and you have a small one. How cool is it that all our bodies are different?' The parents and siblings agreed, and repeated the message that it's cool that our bodies are different. It was a great moment. And that is where we see a shift to a neutral approach not just to your own body, but toward other bodies too."

Eating intuitively

I primarily follow the principles of intuitive eating. In short, this is about eating when you're hungry, stopping when you're full, finding foods that feel good, and not letting what you eat dictate your life. Our bodies hold so much wisdom and can be trusted to eat what they need in the right quantity. "Kids are born as intuitive eaters. There are caveats with genetic issues which might make them struggle to listen to their internal cues, but most healthy children are born knowing what their bodies need nutritionally," explains Megan. "If we have had issues with our own relationships with food, it can be healing to have a child, because you see from the beginning how they are guided by what their body is telling them."

Babies cry when they are hungry and refuse food when they are full. If a baby continues to drink from the bottle a little longer one day, we don't give the baby a lecture on their calorie intake. We let them eat, because the baby is hungry and we don't want them to go hungry. It always boggles my mind how we trust infants with this but we have such a hard time trusting ourselves. Often we restrict our food intake even when we are hungry, but hunger is one of our body's first survival cues.

An approach to feeding kids based on the principles of intuitive eating is baby-led weaning, a method of introducing solid food to babies in which a baby self-feeds. The idea is that it empowers kids and allows them some level of autonomy over food, which is the bedrock for a more in-tune, less shame-driven relationship with their body. Rather than someone else controlling each bite, babies choose how much they want to eat and what they want to eat while they are learning to chew and swallow. "The way we teach baby-led weaning is very flexible. We know it doesn't work for everyone 100 percent, but we want to encourage self-feeding as much as possible," says Megan.

Baby-led weaning is not the only way to feed a kid—at the end of the day, the best baby is a fed baby—and it's not an instant fix for all future food issues, but it is interesting to look at the research behind why we started feeding purees. "The wildest part of my research on infant feeding is how extraordinarily little of our apparently tried-and-tested official advice is based in science," Megan continues. "When I was in college, I believed that the way we introduced baby food was based on some long-established research. But then when I began digging into the literature, I found precisely zero research which supported this pattern of weaning being necessary for babies to learn how to eat. Every single study will mention that infant feeding follows this pattern 'by tradition,' or else they will describe it as 'typical' or 'by custom.' There wasn't any scientific logic and I was alarmed. Why are we doing this?"

As I prepare to become a parent, I've enjoyed researching all things related to kids and food. I follow several parenting food blogs such as Feeding Littles, Solid Starts, Kids Eat in Color, and more. I may not know a thing about strollers or cribs yet, but I have a handful of recipes to try on a toddler (while fully knowing that when I become a parent, my biggest teacher will be my kids). What I've been surprised to find is how much this research has helped me with my own eating. I suppose that's why I wanted to include all of this information here—I don't expect that everyone reading this will be interested in the topic of weaning, but learning about positive feeding techniques for babies and children has helped me with positive feeding techniques for myself.

To give an example, one suggestion for young "picky" eaters is to have them be part of the grocery shopping process, to cook with them, and even have them help in the garden, to expose them to as wide a range of food as possible. I know I'm 99 percent more likely to eat what is in the fridge if I had a hand in choosing it. Recently I've been growing veggies in a small patio garden, and I have never enjoyed eating tomatoes so much. Because I've worked hard to disassociate foods with being "good" or "bad," I now have more options to choose from as I allow myself to respond to my body's hunger cues. It turns out, my sugar cravings were mostly due to not eating enough fat throughout the day.

Another tool I've hijacked from the "picky eater" handbook is to not overwhelm your plate. Especially when faced with a new food or something you don't care for, putting just a tiny little bit on the plate will make it feel less scary and encourage you to actually try it. This was vital for me during my eating disorder recovery. I would often feel sick before I started eating, but having just a little bit allowed me to stomach what was on my plate and encouraged me to have seconds and thirds. It helped me nourish myself better and build up my appetite and palate.

"We've all been trained that if we don't eat this one perfect way, we can't thrive, but there are many ways for kids to grow and thrive," reflects Megan. "We can raise kids with the knowledge that people have all different ideas about food and eating, but in our house, in our family, we listen to our bodies. We don't count calories; we don't omit foods or food groups just because we are trying to change or shrink our bodies. We celebrate our capabilities, whatever those are, and we celebrate the differences in our bodies. We can teach them that, yes, they are going to hear messages that are different to this out there. But this is what *we* do. These kinds of values can really arm them with tools to face the challenges outside of the home." I find Megan's words incredibly encouraging. And what she's describing won't only help those in households with children; it can help all of us to change our attitudes to eating and food.

Finding the confidence to move beyond the "picky eater" label—a label that was applied to me nearly thirty-five years ago—has helped me deal with food anxiety, and allowed me to tune in to my body and find joy in my meals. I may still not enjoy cooking, but I do love eating more than ever before. My eyes have been opened to the ways in which our environment, at home and beyond, can have a fundamental impact on our relationships with food and our bodies—something which I hope will help me fulfill my supposed destiny and break the chain for the next generation.

CHAPTER 5

Neutral Movement

It started with movement

If you had told my younger self that I would have a career in fitness, I would have laughed in your face. Teaching workouts? Not in a million years. But skip to early 2009, the recession was in full swing and no one was hiring. When I got a call back to manage and instruct classes at a new workout studio, I showed up, got the job, and the following day I was taking my first certification class without a clue as to what kind of workout I'd be teaching or if I'd even be good at it. When I think about this time, I'm astounded at how randomly I fell into this career, and how big of an impact it would have on my life, my health, and my happiness—for better and for worse.

Working as a fitness instructor became a mask disguising what was really going on in my personal life. My new studio job was extremely toxic: I worked seven days a week, more than twelve hours a day, with an unstable boss who didn't have my best interests at heart. Then I went home to an abusive romantic relationship fueled by drugs and arguments. Wearing the title of "lead

fitness instructor" at the hot new boutique studio put
a fake gloss over my life and became a reason to excuse
my damaging behaviors. I started eating less and less,
and taking Adderall more and more. I smoked cigarettes
endlessly, and worked out way too many hours each day.
I lived on coffee and Rice Krispies Treats. I threw up
all other meals. I got dizzy so often, my favorite spot to
teach was by the ballet bar so I had something to hold
on to. I was incredibly ill and yet I was praised for my
toned muscles and six-pack.

One of the reasons I'm so adamant about not com-
menting on people's bodies—including their weight
loss—is because you never know what measures someone is taking to look that way. I wish I had heard less
"you look amazing" and more "hey, are you okay?" I
wonder if it would have helped me find recovery faster.
Instead, I was photographed and pinned on the wall as
an example of what our clients should strive to be. To
this day I'm ashamed of the lies I told about what an
attainable body is.

There may have been a lot of darkness then, but there
was also so much light. It was during this time I realized

my strengths and my passion for instructing. Even though I was struggling internally, I have sweet memories associated with the people I met through the studio, many of whom I'm still friends with today. The heart of movement—the body exploration, the routine creation—has always served me. It's my art. And once I began to reframe my workouts, once I put the focus on how I felt, not how I looked, everything changed. Through movement I have healed injuries that plagued me for years; I've gained a better understanding of the mechanics of my body and how it functions; I've become more intuitive when it comes to my body's innate needs and physical desires. I've also strengthened my core, opened my hips, and aligned my neck. I've learned to stand taller and take up space. I've had the chance to marvel at my fingers and toes and the energy I can evoke from the tips of my appendages. Through movement I've released emotions, ignited emotions, and channeled emotions. I learned to teach, gained deep connections with others, and started my business. At this point, it's my life's work, and finding a neutral—even joyful— approach has changed everything for me, in terms of my career, my self-worth, and all of my relationships.

In some ways, this chapter is the reason I'm writing this book. For me, it all started with movement. Throughout my journey, I have learned that movement in and of itself is neutral—it isn't good or bad. The capacity to walk, extend, stretch, contract, wiggle, lift, and pull is function, not value. It's actually one of the reasons you'll notice I tend to use the word "movement" over "exercise" or "workout." Not that there's anything wrong with those words—and no, you don't need to cancel them from your vocabulary—but perhaps renaming them could help you reframe them? To me a "workout" is a set amount of time, at a place that resembles a gym, filled with lunges and squats. To me, "exercise" involves wearing leggings and twisting my body into stretchy positions or counting the number of reps and feeling the burn. But "movement" encompasses so much more, and it does so in a way that respects my body. Movement is dancing in the living room in my underwear, taking a walk with my dogs, swimming in the pool with my nieces and nephews, rolling my head to release my neck after a stressful day. *And* it's going to the gym, squatting, lunging, throwing on my leggings and counting reps. And for you, it may mean something entirely different: movement is a self-expression that is unique and individual to each person. All movement, big or small, long or short, is valid.

What is neutral movement?

When you separate exercise from having the sole goal of changing your body, and instead allow it to be a place for repair, release, and rejuvenation, it's likely you'll find new freedom in your movement practice. In fact, this reframing of how we approach movement is so powerful that it's been given a name—multiple names!—which we will use to guide our conversation in this chapter.

You may or may not have come across the most popular of these, which is the term "joyful movement." (And no, it doesn't mean you run around the gym screaming, "Yippee! I love it here!") Joyful movement emphasizes moving your body in ways that feel good and that you actually enjoy. By decoupling movement from calories lost, movement stops being militant and becomes more free. Other words that have started to pop up around these practices include "intuitive movement" or "intentional movement"—but personally I love the term "neutral movement" (surprise surprise), as it removes expectation or judgment. They all channel the same energy as joyful movement in that none of them involve forced workouts, rigorous calorie counting, or pushing your body where it doesn't want to go. Instead, they are about mindset: movement for the sake of how you feel, not how you look.

My favorite part of neutral movement is that there is an underlying message of body trust. Our bodies are incredibly wise; they know how to adapt, evolve, and even heal themselves. They know when we need rest, and they know when we need to move. As you connect with your body more intuitively, you will be able to interpret its cues in a new way. Aside from helping build strength, movement can also show us our weaknesses, which can help prevent and correct injury. We may notice tight hips, and this encourages us to practice opening the hips and therefore alleviate back pain; or movement may highlight a weakness in our knee joints and signal that we need to strengthen our glutes to support them.

From an emotional perspective, movement can offer support and space for us to release what we have built up inside. Whether that is anger, frustration, pent-up energy, excess energy, sadness, or any other deep feeling, movement can help us shift internal energy, leading to a clearer mind. If you are craving connection, maybe it means working out with a friend or playing with your kids—movement can be a wonderful way to engage with others. From a purely physical point of view, movement can help us take up space: many exercises require sure steps, long arms, big expressions. It can also help channel confidence. Have you ever tried to balance when you're feeling timid? It's much harder than when you're feeling confident. There is so much potential waiting to be unlocked.

What neutral movement is guiding you to do is connect back with your primal self as you discover what type of movement makes you tick. Which exercises feel great for your body, and which types of workouts best serve you? In what ways do you enjoy incorporating activity into your life, and how can you inject more of that daily? Neutral movement is not asking you to stop going to your spin class and it's not asking you to throw away your step tracker. It's asking you to evaluate these tools and activities and determine if they are serving you or hindering you.

Get curious about movement

In my past life, I would have "pushed through" intense movement, no matter what my body told me. I would have believed that it was all a question of mindset and that if I was strong enough, dedicated enough, and "good" enough, I would get through a class or do that run I was forcing myself to do—even if I was sick or exhausted, or generally not functioning well on a phys-ical level.

I still think about the ways I used to speak to myself. I remember going for a run while living in Los Angeles. You should know that I absolutely hate running, but I always felt I should run because runners had thin legs and lithe bodies and so much stamina. One evening, as

I set out, I can remember yelling at my legs: as I hit the pavement with each stride, ringing in my head was *stupid legs, I hate you legs, get skinnier legs, get skinnier, get skinnier!* I thought if I focused all my attention on how disgusting my legs were, I would surely run them away. That's what working out was for me the majority of the time: I would put my mind into my muscles and fill them with nasty thoughts because I believed that this would help my body change faster. This kind of self-talk is part of an abusive relationship that we enter into with ourselves.

One of the best things you can do to shift a toxic relationship with movement is to get curious. Checking in with yourself can be an effective way to discover how movement is currently serving you. In the three steps of the body neutral journey—acknowledge, explore, reconnect—this is the first step: acknowledge. While the experience will be different for everyone, I find it can be helpful to spend some time asking yourself questions and giving honest answers to help you evaluate where you're at.

Next time you do a movement session, try this mindful exercise:

Am I ... ?

- Feeling connected to my body?
- Enjoying the release of emotion?
- Appreciating the functions of my body without criticism?
- Able to identify areas of tightness, flexibility, pain, and strength?
- Listening to and honoring my body's needs?
- Moving without judgment or set expectations?

When we are able to answer yes to these questions, we are on track for participating in neutral movement. On the flip side you may notice that your mindset is less than neutral. Ask yourself these questions:

Am I ... ?

- Focused on my body's failings?
- Concentrating on the amount of time spent in movement rather than how my body feels?
- Disappointed/hard on myself when I cannot achieve a certain position variation?

- Comparing myself to others?
- Labeling my movement as "good" vs. "bad"?
- Pushing my body dangerously past its limits for the sake of hitting a certain goal/target?

If you find yourself answering yes to second set of questions, taking a step back could prove beneficial. Over time, this way of thinking can be detrimental not only to your physical health (injuries and pain), but also to your mental outlook (body dysmorphia, exercise abuse).

Don't be surprised if your answers to the questions aren't cut and dried. Maybe you're enjoying the release of emotion and marveling at all the functions of your body while also mad as hell that you dropped out of the plank. Both can be true at the same time! The goal is to move toward a more neutral way of thinking while taking the pressure off yourself to be perfect. And honestly, try to have some fun in the meantime. Getting to move your body around should be, for the most part, enjoyable. But it will likely take time to get to a neutral perspective—and like anything, you'll experience days that are easier than others.

Maybe checking in with yourself during movement feels like too much pressure. After all, it can be nice to turn your brain *off* during this time. If that's the case, try spending a few minutes before and/or after your session checking in with yourself. Try asking yourself some or all of the following questions, depending on the day:

Questions to ask yourself pre-movement

Why am I choosing to move today? Is it based on changing my physical form? If yes, can I reframe my motive for this movement session to focus on my mental, spiritual, or emotional self?

How are my energy levels? Am I in need of restorative movement or energetic movement?

Where am I experiencing tightness? Would stretching my back/neck/legs/hips serve me? What can I do during my movement session to promote healing?

What is one thing I'm grateful for that my body can do?

How do I want this movement session to serve me?

Questions to ask yourself post-movement

In what ways did I listen to my body in this movement session? How can I better listen to my body in future movement sessions?

How did my movement affect my mood today?

How are my energy levels? Do I feel more tired or more energized?

Where am I experiencing tightness in my body? Do I need to do any restorative practices today such as taking a bath, icing, or stretching?

In what ways did my body show up for me in this session?

Did I enjoy the movement I just did? Why or why not? Is this a type of movement I will show up to again?

Getting curious about the workouts we engage in, the exercises we do, and the movement we choose to participate in can help us inject more joy into our lives. That may sound like a lofty promise, but it's the truth. Maybe you truly love strength-training classes and enjoy lifting a kettlebell over your head. But maybe you don't enjoy it at all. Maybe you have always hated lifting weights but you put yourself through it because you've been told you have to in order to look/feel/be a certain way. It's only when you take the time to question yourself deeply and without judgment that you're able to discover your own answers. And why spend precious moments of your life doing something you hate? There are endless ways to move and explore your body, and life is too short to be grinding through a fitness class that brings you zero joy. It's time to recalibrate and let your body be in charge.

Explore your movement prejudices

Up until a certain age, or until someone tells them otherwise, kids participate in movement because it's fun, not because it's necessary. They don't care what they look like when on the swings, and don't notice if they make strange faces or sounds when jumping on the trampoline. They certainly aren't thinking about their form or calories burned when running across the playground. They just want to move, and at school they live for recess. They only begin to think about movement as a means to change their body when they receive messages that their bodies need to change. It is learned behavior, not inherent behavior.

These messages are often associated with an idea best described as the "morality of exercise." Over time, a fit body became part of the American dream, and with that came hundreds of thousands of gyms and a multibillion-dollar industry. The hour-long fitness class, the five-times-a-week rule, 10,000 steps a day, all became more than suggestions—they became the only path to a good life. I'm not saying counting your steps is evil. I do believe that more activity would serve many of us in terms of our overall well-being, and I get it, we want to preserve our bodies and thrive. But the media's tactics are all so fear-based and don't put the wisdom and autonomy of our bodies at the forefront. Simply put, spending thirty minutes on the treadmill does not make you a better person. What makes you a better person is treating others with kindness and giving all people—regardless of looks, status, race, gender, wealth, ability—appreciation and respect. Maybe this feels obvious to you, but fear-based messaging follows us throughout our lives. Read any pregnancy advice platform, and they'll make you feel like the worst parent-to-be if you're not exercising for thirty minutes every single day.

A myth that works against our body's autonomy is the idea that we can't motivate ourselves to move without guilting ourselves to go to the gym or shaming our body into a workout class. In an exercise class, for example, instructors might say things like "If anyone drops out of their plank, we are all starting over!" Sure, that is a motivator. Who wants to start a plank over? And this kind of language isn't an instructor's fault—it is likely how they've been trained. However, motivators like this don't encourage you to tune in to your body and they don't create a long-lasting relationship with movement. Either you'll injure yourself and then you can't plank at all, or you'll begin to associate planks with shame.

A more helpful form of motivation is one that asks us to get curious about our bodies: "What does it feel like if you get lower in your squat? Do you feel it more in your butt or less?" If you heard this in class, you might be tempted to test your range of motion and determine what squat height is right for you.

At this point, I want to invite you to think about the external factors that are influencing your approach to movement. Here are some questions that can help you get curious:

How did movement play out in your childhood? What activities did you enjoy? What activities did you dislike? Why?

Do you have any adolescent memories—good or bad—that come up when you think of movement and exercise?

How did your parents/guardians or elders approach exercise? In what ways do you see these practices show up in your life?

When you think of the word "exercise," name the first five words that come to mind. When or where did you begin to associate these words with exercise?

What kind of language does your instructor use in your workout classes? What kind of language does your gym promote? Is this language in line with your values?

Who influences your approach to movement either online or in real life? Do their values support your body neutral journey?

What do you consume that frames exercise as a punishment, a requirement, or a means only to change your physical shape? What do you consume that frames exercise as a treat, a healing modality, or a means to better your mind/body/spirit?

Once you are able to identify where your prejudices about movement are coming from, you can then work to reconnect with your movement practice.

All movement is valid

Over the years, the motto "All movement is valid" has supported my journey and helped me find what neutral movement looks like in my life. I used to rate my workouts based on calories burned, time spent, sweat dripped, and soreness of muscles the next day, but movement is so much more than this. Did you walk up the stairs instead of taking the elevator? Did you carry a child on your back or in a sling for part of the day? Did you sprint for the bus, or to catch your dog at the park? Did you pack boxes, tend to the garden, or bend to the ground a hundred times doing laundry? Playing on the floor with your kids is movement. Commuting is movement. Climbing stairs is movement. You do not need to be in your workout clothes for it to count.

The benefit of viewing all movement as valid is that it can be a big step in thinking of movement in more neutral terms. We tend to be less judgmental of our activities outside of our workout environment. For example, I find it easy to judge my performance on the treadmill or in the weight room, but I never think, *I could have commuted better.* I'm sure most parents reading have never thought, *I could have put more effort into playing horsey with my four-year-old.* Or, *I should have lifted my 21-pound toddler 15 percent higher.* As we work to release ingrained ideas of the "good workout" and "bad workout," let's connect with the simple movements that fill and enrich our lives daily.

A good way to do this is to think back to your childhood, before the concept of workouts entered your psyche. What was your go-to activity? Swimming? Tag? Four square? A dance party? Think about all the things you loved to do and note them down. Now, looking at your list, do any of these activities still make you smile? Do any of them sound appealing or fun? If so, how could you incorporate them into your daily life now? What about your friends—could you enlist people in your life to embark on a group activity? Backyard volleyball, couples' tennis, sledding, frisbee golf, softball, even a rousing game of charades: not only will you get your body moving, you'll cultivate community and make some awesome memories in the process.

When I was a kid, I really liked to jump rope, so a couple of years ago I got a jump rope and started jumping my way down the street. Now, I've taken workout classes that involved a jump rope and I hated them. Yet when I remembered my love of jumping rope as a kid, and approached the exercise in that manner, I had an absolute blast! Why? Because I didn't need to keep to a rhythm of one minute on and thirty seconds off. I didn't have to jump to a certain beat or at a certain speed. Little kid Bethany just hopped down the street to her heart's desire. It was freeing, fun, and childlike—and completely neutral. And my favorite playground activity? The swings. I spent hours on the swings as a kid. So, over the summer, my jump rope and I made our way to a local playground and swung on the swings. I swear, I smiled the *entire* time, and yes, that was my workout for the day.

All movement, silly or serious, hard or easy, functional or fun, is valid movement. Working to internalize this and find new ways to move your body can help you form a better relationship with movement. When you put your body and your needs first, whatever shows up is what you needed that day. Remember, your body is wise beyond belief, and you are a living miracle. Trust yourself as you embark upon your neutral movement journey.

Change your intent

One of the most powerful tools that can help in accepting that all movement is valid is taking a step back and homing in on your personal reasons for moving in the first place. There are the so-called objective and health-based ones, such as regular exercise helping to prevent chronic illness and premature death—and a lot of money has gone into research proving that movement extends your life span and your quality of life. However, it's important to remember that you could follow every single rule and live like a monk and still not make it to a hundred. I'm not going to guilt you into getting in x minutes of movement a week or eating five portions of fruit and veg a day, or avoiding more than one glass of wine, or whatever it is the current batch of studies are prescribing. That's not what this book is about.

Instead, I'm going to ask you how you feel when you *don't* move. During the period when I was healing from my eating disorders, I decided to do an experiment to help shift my relationship with exercise. Whenever I wanted to do any dedicated movement, I only allowed myself to do it if I could find a reason beyond making body changes. I would ask myself, *What's the reason I want to work out today?* At first, it was physical every single time: *I'm so bloated, I ate too much last night, I need to tone up my legs* . . . I couldn't find a reason beyond the physical, and so I'd stay home.

The longer I didn't exercise, the more my motivation began to shift. I started to feel itchy, trapped, stagnant. Soon I didn't care if I was bloated, or if I had eaten "too much"; I just needed a release, to clear my head, to feel my heart beat in my chest. My body wanted to feel a burst of endorphins, to jolt it out of inertia. I longed for activity—not to get a six-pack, but because my wise physical self knew it was ready for action.

In this process, give yourself grace and remember that it is okay to have days when you are not motivated and it is okay to take time off. There have been times when my wise physical self knew it needed to rest and wasn't interested in movement at all—like when I was going through fertility treatment. The hormonal overload made me feel lethargic, and the only thing that felt good was gentle walking. But the key here is that, by getting in touch with my body, I was able to listen to its cues and respect its needs. It goes without saying that during times of crisis—be that grieving, going through a breakup, struggling with mental health, or just having a difficult time—movement might not be your priority. Equally, for some people, a workout could offer solace in dark times. There aren't any universal rules on how movement can support and enhance your life.

Soon, you will notice what a difference reframing your movement motivations can make, and how it can help in creating a sustainable relationship with movement. It's less about "I *have* to go to the gym" and more about "I *get* to be active today." Once movement (in any form) becomes a way for you to express, explore, and experiment, it can become a fun place rather than a dreadful one. I've always been curious about motivation in general, so over the years I've polled my clients, asking what helps them feel motivated. Here are some of their answers which you can use for some shame-free, non-physical motivation.

Think about ...

How it will feel after: "I think about the feeling afterward and how amazing it can feel to move without judgment. Letting go of the idea of movement as punishment allows me to focus on what feels good for my body, and those sensations can be a great motivator!"

Movement as a powerful release: "Honestly, today what motivated me was the shitty day I had. Some air punching was a good I-need-to-hit-something release."

Movement as self-care: "Life is unpredictable . . . And some days, it's too much. Movement gives me a beautiful, grounding reorientation to the present, to my body, to my brain, exactly as they are, right now. When I'm heading to a dark place, it saves me."

Create an atmosphere: "I find it so calming to move at 5am, lights off, eyes closed (mostly), enjoying the music. I light some candles, burn some incense, and make my room serve boutique studio realness."

Listen to your body

Have you ever watched a bee when it's raining? They can't fly in the rain so they hide under leaves while they wait out the storm before continuing to do their work. If you've ever felt like a bee, you're not alone. The majority of nature takes a snooze before spring—trees, flowers, grass, hibernating animals, you name it. I used to be really hard on myself when the weather affected my workout—how dare I spend this rainy day with a movie on the couch instead of pounding it out at the gym!—but I've learned to lean into the idea that nature ebbs and flows and so do I. Flowers are not always in bloom, the moon is not always full, and the tide is not always high. Our capacity and enthusiasm for movement fluctuates, and some days are made for rest.

When you've been conditioned to believe that you should be active 100 percent of the time, it's normal to find it difficult to read your body's cues and distinguish whether your mood is low and you need to restore, or your mood is low and you need to get moving. The ability to listen to our innate cues is a muscle we can flex and strengthen. Here are some signs that could help you decide if today is a movement day or a rest day, though it goes without saying that you know your body best!

Signs your body may be craving movement:

- lethargy
- boredom
- foggy mind/forgetfulness
- body feels tight or stiff
- overstimulated
- struggling to fall asleep
- pent-up energy
- restlessness
- constipation
- cold body temperature
- a desire to refresh

Signs your body may be craving rest:

- sore muscles
- joint pain/injury

- cramping/muscle fatigue
- exhaustion
- overstressed or working long hours
- emotional distress
- heavy menstrual flow
- a life event that requires attention
- a desire to restore
- your workout feels harder than normal

If you find yourself struggling to decide if movement is what you need—maybe the line between "lethargy" and "exhaustion" feels blurry—I recommend starting small. Take a walk around the block, or sit on a mat and stretch for five minutes. It may be a nice time to ask yourself some of the questions we talked about on pages 134–5. Close your eyes, touch your body, breathe deeply. Notice if you slightly rock forward (often an internal sign of "yes") or if you rock back (often an internal sign of "no"). Let your body be the decision-maker. You may find you end up doing a long workout and enjoying every minute of it; you may also find that five minutes of stretching is your exercise for the day. It's not about telling yourself you're going to just do a little, but when you get there, you're actually going to do it all, *right*? No. Give yourself permission to make it small. It will make it easier to reconnect with yourself, tune in to your desires, and empower your body.

When I left studio life to launch the be.come project, giving my clients the power to make decisions about their bodies was of the utmost importance. One of the things I work hard to do is take away the virtue of a move—for example, not saying that doing a plank on your knees is "bad" and that doing a plank on your feet is "good." With any exercise, the hardest version is the one in which you feel it in all the right spots because this is the position where your muscles are working the hardest. If that means you do your plank off a wall, then so be it. As an instructor, I encourage clients to explore the position that works best for them without placing any value on the action. In fact, I've stopped using the word "modification" because it implies "easier"; I prefer "alternative" because it is simply something different. Words go a long way in a fitness class.

1. Go for a walk with a purpose.

a) **Focus on your surroundings to help you recenter.** Before you set out, close your eyes and think of a color—whichever color comes to your mind first. As you walk, see how many times you spot this color and where, and how many variations on the shade you notice.

b) **Get your blood moving with a brisk walk.** Try quickening your pace without forcing anything. It may help to listen to an energetic playlist and see how it feels to keep pace with the tempo of the music.

c) **Concentrate on deep breathing as you walk.** Ignore your pace completely and just listen to your breath as you walk. Try taking slow, audible inhales and exhales, or if you want something more structured, search "guided breathing" on YouTube!

d) **Try a walk/workout combo.** Experiment with movement you can add to your walk. Perhaps it's a few minutes of jump rope. Maybe at the end of each song on your playlist you stop to do ten squats. Why not try a few push-ups off a wall every three blocks? You could see if walking lunges feel right for your body, or even explore wearing ankle or wrist weights.

e) **Use your walk to escape!** Walk on a treadmill or elliptical and watch your favorite TV show. Perhaps on this day, you don't need mindful movement—maybe you need some mindless movement! If you're craving both an escape and some activity, walk indoors and enjoy some screen time.

2. Simple stretching—never underestimate the power of a stretch! Here are some simple poses that can help you release and restore:

Forward fold with cradle arms: Stand with feet hip-width apart, knees soft. Let your upper body dangle to the floor. Grab either elbow to make a "cradle" with your arms and let your head hang heavy.

Seated figure-four hip stretch: Sit on a chair. Bring one ankle up to the opposite knee so that your leg makes a "figure 4" shape and relaxes open. Option to lean the upper body forward.

Seated wide-leg forward fold: Sit on the floor, on a pillow, or on a block. Open your legs to a comfortable "V" position. Hold here or lean forward. Try gently swaying side to side.

Squeeze and release: Exhale and squeeze your hands into fists, hold for one count. Release your hands and inhale deeply. Repeat.

Posture reset: Stand with feet hip-width apart. Turn your palms to face backward and move your arms slightly behind your body. Bring your thumbs closer together. You should feel your chest opening.

Butterfly stretch: Sit on the floor, on a pillow, or on a block. Bring the soles of your feet together so your legs form a "butterfly" shape. Allow your knees to fall open, let your hips and stomach relax. Option to lean your upper body forward.

Standing breath: Stand with feet hip-width apart and rooted. Turn palms forward, roll your shoulders, gently lift your heart. Inhale and then slowly exhale.

Legs up against a wall: Lay on the floor with your butt close to a wall. Put your legs up against the wall so that your feet are facing up. Let your legs stay soft and don't force the position.

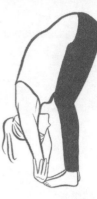

forward fold with cradle arms

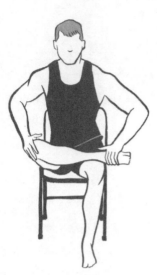

seated figure-four hip stretch

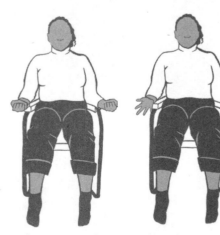

seated wide-leg forward fold

squeeze and release

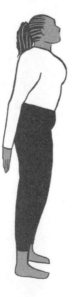

posture reset

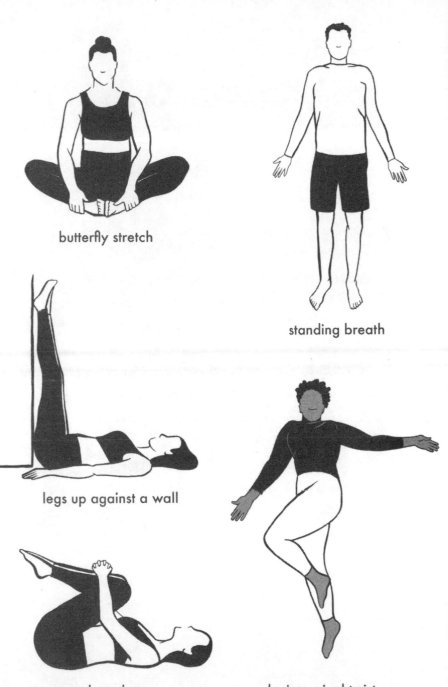

butterfly stretch

standing breath

legs up against a wall

laying spinal twist

knee hug

Knee hug: Lay on the ground. Bring both knees into your chest and wrap your arms around your legs. Give them a hug as you relax your head to the floor. If your arms don't reach, try holding a towel or strap to give you extra length.

Laying spinal twist: Lay on the ground with legs extended. Bring one knee to your chest and gently guide it across your body, so that your lower half is twisted. Let the arms fall to a "T" position. For more support, place a pillow under the twisting leg.

3. Feeling energized but don't have a lot of time?
Choose an energetic song (3–4 minutes) and try doing these moves! Stay in each move for as long as your body wants, and repeat as many times as you like.

- quick punches
- squats
- plank holds

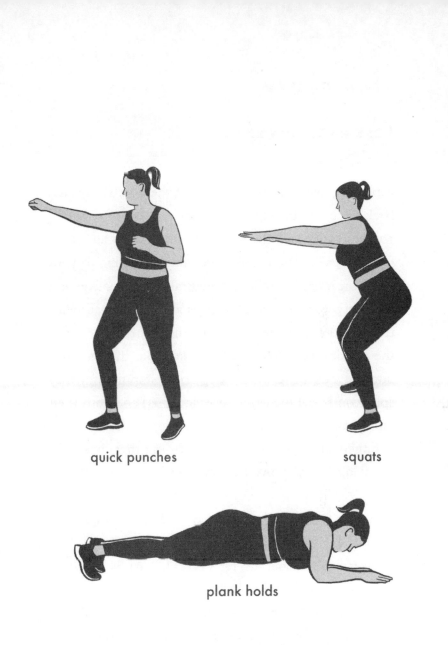

quick punches

squats

plank holds

Let's move forward

One thing I've noticed since launching the be.come project is that whatever I put out there gets repeated back to me by my clients. The more I express that all movement is valid, the more my clients treat all movement as valid. The more I encourage listening to your body, the more I see clients freely taking alternatives and mindful breaks. The more I speak about body neutrality, the more I notice clients shifting their worth away from the physical self. Not only do I see it in the way they interact with themselves, I also notice it in the way they speak on social media, with each other, and with their family members. I want to share some of my favorite comments here, so you can hear from others how life-changing neutral movement can be:

> I have chronic pain, and I have a deal with myself that if I feel up to movement, I'll do it. If not, I won't worry about it. This week I haven't felt up to it, and discovered that the body neutral movement of be.come really supports my plan. No shame, no judgment about not being up to it. It makes it so much

easier to return to movement when I feel better! Feeling grateful about that.

—Zoe G.

Oh, the message at the end of this week's routine hit the core for me. I felt so bad about not being good at exercising but this is a new attempt and I need to meet myself where I am right now. I find it hard to trust my body because of lack of exercise, but I will grow into it. All movement is valid, that's totally it.

—Rüveyda Soyupak

I really appreciated your message of body autonomy. I cried after this and it felt so moving to be given these reminders in such loving and compassionate ways while moving, listening to, and caring for my body (whilst in therapy from sexual trauma—I'm trying to listen and respect my body's knowing and often feel defeated/it's impossible). This felt so hopeful. Thank you so much—it felt like a cathartic practice in so many ways.

—Alex Balfour

I took a workout class recently and it wasn't my typical class. The instructor talked about flattening our stomachs and toning our thighs and laid on a guilt trip for what we ate over the weekend. But believe it or not, it served as a wonderful reminder of where I have been and where I am now. I reframed the instructor's words to suit me—*this move will prevent lower back pain, this one is opening my hips, I can feel my glutes activating here.* I chose alternatives, moved my push-ups to a wall, asked for blocks, and moved at my own pace. While in the past I would have felt embarrassed, now I felt powerful. Mentally reframing the class from a more neutral standpoint allowed me to connect with myself, connect with my friends in the class, and enjoy the movement at hand. In fact, during the class I noticed some other people taking the same alternatives I did. And after the class my friends and I had a riveting discussion where we ended up agreeing that the "flatten your stomach" talk during a workout feels outdated.

The fitness world is not all bad. Sure, I've taken classes and encountered spaces that have made me feel bad about myself. But I have also been in classes which have left me feeling empowered, supported, and uplifted. At the end of the day, I have found more joy through movement than I have sadness, even if I had to create that joy myself. When we think about movement as a way to release and improve how our body functions, not just a way to lose weight or drop a dress size, it can be incredibly empowering. We are all trying to figure it out, and some will get there faster than others and that's okay. What my experience has taught me is that we all have the power to be the light for ourselves, and then shine it on others too.

CHAPTER 6

Let It Go

The control myth

I have a love-hate relationship with the advice to "let it go." In some ways, I love its simplicity. I love the idea of all my cares melting off my shoulders and forming a puddle beneath me, while I delicately leap my way over the muck and waltz off into the sunshine a new person. But I also hate how simple it is because it's almost offensive: like when you're upset and someone tells you to "calm down." Or when you're struggling to get pregnant and someone tells you to "stop trying." Or when you're feeling anxious and someone suggests "just relax." Listen to me when I say that if I knew how to "let go" of all my neuroses, I happily would have by now!

The desire to be in control can play a big part in how we treat our bodies. This is because we've been sold a myth—the myth that what we look like is within our sole power to control, and that if we don't like what we see in the mirror, it is up to us to change it. We might push our bodies to extremes to try to be something other than what we are, and end up feeling unhappy and vulnerable. Sometimes, we even put our well-being in danger, undernourishing ourselves in an effort to be thin. Or pumping ourselves with artificial steroids to develop Superman-like muscles.

And what's worse is it doesn't stop at our physical appearance. Time and time again, on social media and in popular self-help books, we are told that "we all have the same twenty-four hours" and that if we're not living our dream life, it's because we haven't tried hard enough. But this idea fails to acknowledge that, while there is a lot that we can do to create a life that fulfills us, there will always be things that are beyond our control—whether that's an unexpected illness, losing a loved one, being laid off from a job, or the life and family that we are born into. Instead of finding a way to accept that this is an inevitable part of life, we are taught that we must control everything about ourselves, when really it's that lie that is controlling us.

I now realize that I used to—and probably still do—internalize this lie, which for me manifested as a deep desire to control all aspects of myself. This is in part what led me to addictive and damaging behaviors. My eating disorder was extremely rooted in control: the more out of control my life was, the more in control I had to be of my body.

Let me explain this using an analogy that might resonate with you. Have you ever been anxiously awaiting news? And in that moment, did you find yourself mindlessly cleaning in order to channel your nerves? You feel out of control waiting for the news, so you resort to something you know you have power over. You may not be able to control the news you are going to receive, but you sure as hell can make that countertop shine. It gives you an illusion of control, and that feels good.

This will inevitably look different for everyone. "If you have a disability or chronic health condition—which is ostensibly a reminder that we cannot truly possess control over the body—I think the challenge of releasing control is about redirection and finding power through another means that doesn't revolve around the body," Lottie Jackson says. "For me, this would be writing, being creative, and getting involved with activism—all of which allow me to express myself and feel a sense of strength in who I am."

Now that I am in recovery, I'm still very fond of activities where I can see the results as I work: painting a wall, mowing the lawn. The satisfaction of visible results really gets me off (in case I needed further proof that I love to be in charge). When the Covid pandemic hit in 2020, I cleaned/painted/gardened as much as I could, to keep my hands busy and gain a sense of control during a time when I felt absolutely powerless—and I'm certain I wasn't alone in that. We see a "lack of control" turning into a "need to control" often, but I don't think it's always a bad thing. In fact, that's my problem with the "let it go" mentality—sometimes, you need that feeling of control, even if you know it's an illusion. The key here is how we channel that energy. Do we put it toward something that is positive and could benefit us, something neutral which could support us, or something negative that could hurt us? How do we find an equilibrium?

When control controls you

While writing this book, most of the conversations I had about body neutrality landed back at the issue of control. When we talk about our bodies, much of the language is wrapped up in self-discipline and our ability to control our size, shape, intake, and output. But many people's journey to healing involves giving up control in some form, as mine did. There's an untrue perception in our society that slimmer, smaller people are more put together—mainly because they are perceived to have more self-control. But paradoxically, what I have learned is that when we try to overly control anything in our life, it ends up controlling us, leaving us anything but put together.

An excessive desire for control can swing our personal pendulum in extreme directions, taking us on a path to self-destruction. In the context of the body, the more we try to control what we eat, how we exercise, and how our outer self appears to the world, the more these issues will loom large in our life, depleting our health and happiness.

When I think of excessive control in my own life, I go back to the time I was a raw foodist. It was shortly after I had moved to Chicago, my first big city, and during a time when I was figuring myself out—exploring myself and my beliefs outside of the rigid environment of my small-town life. I was lost and seeking structure, and raw foodism offered me that structure. Now I can see that I was just replacing one extreme way of life with another. The lifestyle involves eating only uncooked fruits, vegetables, and nuts; you eat nothing cooked, refined, pasteurized, or processed. Basically, imagine a bunny rabbit diet, and that's raw foodism. I found comfort in the lofty promises, rules, and culture, and it became my new religion. For a while, it was amazing—I felt better, stronger, and more powerful than ever—but like most things we do for the wrong reasons, that quickly faded and developed into one of the early markers of my eating disorders.

The high I got from eating raw was completely based on a perceived ability to control my life. I didn't need restaurants or get-togethers or fancy cookware. I was above that, and I judged everyone who did need it. What I didn't realize is what I was missing out on: I missed out on family holidays, I didn't eat my grandparents' delicious meals, I stopped being invited to dinners with friends. I became isolated and alone. I remember feeling like a withering flower, desperate for sustenance.

Johanna Kandel tells me that understanding the role of control was one of the biggest keys to gaining clarity on her relationship with her body. "What I realized was that my eating disorder was giving me an elusive form of control," she explains. "The best I can describe it, it was like I was a really bad backseat driver, where I was the one who I thought was actually driving the car, when actually my eating disorder had both hands on the wheel. For so long I thought that I was in control. But now I'm on the other side, I realize how much of a lack of control I really had, because I hated every minute of my eating disorder, yet I was so scared to live my life without it. Recovery has given me the opportunity to climb over the central console and grab hold of the wheel."

What I now understand is that whatever you restrict becomes the thing you crave. Whenever I inevitably broke the raw food "rules" and ate something cooked, I would throw it up to get it out of my system. In my mind, it was better to purge than it was to eat something not in its raw state. However, two years into this lifestyle, my deep restrictions led to more and more cravings, which led to more and more bingeing, which led to more and more purging. I remember once wanting a donut so badly that it consumed my entire day. I ended up stopping at a bakery and got the donut and ate it in the car, and then, while driving, forced myself to throw it up in the bag. What's worse, I shamed and blamed myself for not being strong enough to fight the craving. That moment was one of my lowest points. In the end, I stopped eating raw, but I was left with these structures of control which led to me turning to drugs and eating disorders I would battle for years. I had become obsessed with the feeling of being in control, of having power over myself, of being "good."

When we spoke, Dr. Pooja Lakshmin gave helpful guidelines for establishing whether or not your desire for control has started to control you. "The moment that your need for control begins to take over your functioning is where I would be concerned. From a clinical perspective, what we mean here is when your functioning starts to change. Perhaps you are turning up late for work, or missing meetings because you can't fit in your food prep or fitness regime. Perhaps you have stopped socializing around food, or you are rearranging your calendar to fit in specific classes, to the detriment of your relationships. The other thing I would question is the guilt factor. When the volume of the self-critical talk and the guilt is so high, it can be very damaging to your overall mental health. That's another place you could draw a line, even if functioning is intact."

Using these guidelines, I want to encourage you to ask yourself some questions about your relationship with control. As with many things, it's not a black-and-white issue, but rather a sliding scale that shifts and changes.

Are your habits impeding upon your everyday life, such as work schedule, time with family, or time with friends?

Do you say no to events/occasions/activities in order to stick to your regimen?

How much are you beating yourself up when you make a misstep? Is it something that becomes quite dramatic?

> Are you someone who is consistently tough on
> yourself?

Loosening the reins

Starting to let go is never going to be an overnight thing. It is going to be a process, and one in which you will likely take small steps. When I was ill with my eating disorder, one of the ways I sought to control my body was to keep the house empty of food. If I wanted chips, I'd have to go out and buy the chips, eat the whole bag, and not have them anymore. Now that I'm in recovery, one of the most important practical steps I have taken is to always make sure the pantry is stocked, and I feel fortunate that this is something I can afford. There are always bars, there are always chips, there are always nuts. And there's always chocolate. Because what I have learned is that the more access I have to it, the less power it has over me. At first, I found doing this incredibly scary. I started by picking one food that was formerly a "no" food to have around, and once that felt safe, I started to add more. Now I'll forget that my favorite snack is even in the cupboard. Buying a bunch of food isn't going to magically cure your disordered eating, but removing restrictions is an important part of the recovery process.

Changing everything at once can feel terrifying, so what if instead of making big dramatic changes, you experimented with modest changes? You can always decide they don't work for you and go back to your previous tack, but why not see what it feels like to loosen the reins from time to time? Making small changes is a great way to move closer to your goal without feeling overwhelmed. Here is a quick exercise to get you going:

Step 1: Write down a few absolutes in your life. Ideally these are hard rules or regimens that don't always serve you or that limit you from certain life situations.

Step 2: What's a small, manageable habit that you can start implementing today to start to loosen the reins? It shouldn't feel like a 180-degree shift, but should be something practical, grounded, and actionable. Start small and get curious!

Step 3: How can you lean on people that you love to support you in this change? Make a list of three people that you can talk to about this change you want to make and who will help you as you put it into practice.

The power of self-compassion

Here's the thing: having some control over our lives can be a really good thing. Self-control—our ability to override short-term temptations and desires that conflict with our long-cherished goals—can help to create structure, which in turn can help us to achieve our dreams. This process can also bring a sense of meaning to our lives. People who display self-control have been shown to be happier, more satisfied, and experience better well-being. They often have better relationships, finances, and more successful careers. These are all obviously great things.

But if you are a control-oriented person, it can be very challenging to have a specific goal in mind and not put all of your energy into trying to achieve it. Perhaps you are studying for a qualification, or trying to be a perfect parent, or attempting to build a new career. In all these instances, self-control could support your goals, but it could also cross the line and become detrimental, leading to burnout or putting you under an unsustainable amount of pressure. It is kind of like recovering from an injury—a few physical therapy exercises will strengthen the muscle, but take it too far with rigorous exercise and you could reinjure yourself. When it comes to control and being compassionate with ourselves, it's all about finding balance.

"The ability to treat yourself with compassion is a struggle for so many of my patients and it is something I have to contend with myself," admits Pooja. "It can be so confronting when the framework you have built your life and success upon is challenged—if self-discipline got you here, surely letting yourself off the hook will undermine everything you have achieved? One thing we can do to help alleviate this fear is to remember that practicing self-compassion is not going to change your personality. At times you are still going to be hard on yourself and that is okay. If you have only ever shamed yourself into productivity and success, it is worthwhile considering if another framework is open to you. Importantly, we can focus not on what we might feel we are 'losing' through letting go of some of our self-discipline, but what we might gain through self-compassion. Yes, you might not be as productive when you are more compassionate with yourself. But opening that space may enable something else into your life and it may be better. We don't know, but it's having this curiosity to see and being okay with that uncertainty."

When I was launching the be.come project, I was incredibly rigid about the date it would go to market. It had to be July 16, *or else*. I remember talking to my therapist at the time about how I *had* to launch July 16, and I also remember being offended when she asked me why. The truth was, I didn't know why. It was the date I had set and I suppose I didn't want to let myself down. I launched on time but I pushed myself to the limit to get there. A few days before, I was in San Francisco with my spouse and I was so pent-up I couldn't enjoy it. I took my computer with me everywhere I went, cried every day, and I even threw my back out. I launched regardless of the state of the platform, and when I did, basically all of my tech broke. I spent the next three months fixing mistakes that probably could have been avoided if I'd just slowed down.

The next time I had a big launch, I decided to switch it up and gave myself a flexible date. I pushed to have it done when I wanted, but I also didn't give up my well-being to make it happen. And you know what? It was a little delayed, but it launched with ease and my team and I were happier and more rested. Becoming compassionate with myself and letting go of arbitrary deadlines allowed me to have a more fulfilled and enjoyable experience. When we speak of balance, self-compassion can help us moderate an excessive need for control.

"One of the biggest lessons I've learned when it comes to control," says Johanna, "is that wanting to control things is okay and natural. The learning has come from *also* allowing myself the space and grace to be a human being. Finding that balance has been so central to my recovery and redefining my relationship with my body and beyond." By not holding ourselves to unrealistic standards or unsustainable regimens, we can be gentler on ourselves and help prevent our pendulum lurching to extremes. If we engage in unkind thoughts or damaging behaviors, we can have compassion and understand that we are operating in a world that doesn't necessarily want us to be content. We can, with grace, step back to acknowledge what might have influenced us to make those decisions and explore those factors calmly. If we feel we have let ourselves down, we can remind ourselves that our bodies, our productivity, everything about us is meant to ebb and flow, and that in nature everything is fluid. Self-control without self-compassion may not only mean you miss out on many of the pleasures of life, it may also alienate you from your true self and all its glories.

As for how this works practically, Pooja emphasizes taking things gently. "I'm definitely not saying you're going to take this Pollyanna approach to talking to yourself, because that would be inauthentic. Instead, it's just trying to dial down the volume of self-criticism. Ask yourself: *Where did this voice come from? Where did I learn this? What would it feel like if I were to be gentle with myself here?* At first, it really might feel like a loss to not be driving yourself so hard, so you have to trust that in that space something new, perhaps more authentic, will come through. But it will take time. Just keep asking yourself those questions to make the shift as tolerable as possible."

When things are out of your control

Even when you know all the steps, it can be a struggle to treat yourself with compassion. Recently I went through an intense experience where a lack of control over my body had a profound impact on my mental and physical health, but I found that leaning into the lessons of body neutrality was one of the best ways I could support myself through it.

I have always known I wanted to be a parent; that has never been a question for me. I equally didn't doubt it would be easy to get pregnant once I decided the time was right. In fact, I would have bet a million dollars that it was going to happen on command, just like clicking my fingers. When I got my period after our first month of trying, my initial reaction was confusion. I had already stocked up on anti-nausea vitamins and pregnancy tests. After two years of IUI cycles, a nonviable pregnancy, miscarriage, prepping for an IVF cycle, egg retrieval, and countless negative results, it's safe to say that my gut instinct was off. In fact, I couldn't have been more wrong, and I felt completely betrayed by my intuition.

It can be very hard to be neutral when you feel your body is letting you down, and with all the will in the world and all the medicine and doctors, you cannot force your body to be pregnant, or cancer-free, or unencumbered by pain. Megan McNamee often sees a similar cycle play out with her clients. "For people who have experienced infertility, or people who have dealt with significant health issues, it is easy to start to lose trust and faith in your body in a lot of ways. There can be a lot of anger toward the body and then a desire to control it. The impulse is often to try and make our bodies do what we want them to do. I work with a lot of people with chronic health issues, and I've had chronic health issues myself, and it's so interesting to see how there becomes this 'Right, you're doing it again, you're letting me down again, I don't have any faith or trust in you anymore.'"

Pooja explains that in instances where you feel let down by your body, it's important to allow yourself to go through the grieving process. "You need to let yourself grieve what your body hasn't been able to give you, or what your body can no longer give you and what you have lost. The acknowledgment piece is so important here, and you have to allow yourself to feel sad. For many people, it can feel scary to confront that grief and accept that there has been a loss, especially when it comes to infertility and miscarriage. There's all this pressure from the outside— the 'don't worry, you'll get pregnant again' or 'it wasn't meant to be.' But letting yourself be sad and finding other people who are able to tolerate being in that sadness with you is your first step toward acceptance. I treat many women dealing with chronic illness or infertility or women who have a child with special needs. In all instances, until they go through a true mourning period for what has been lost, it is impossible to reach a point of neutrality. You can't skip that step."

The month I turned thirty-five also marked the sixth month of us trying to conceive, and it brought me to my knees with grief. Even though six months isn't long to be trying for a baby, it hit me hard. The morning I started my period, I walked outside and found a dead bird in my yard. In fact, I encountered three dead birds on days my period started throughout our journey trying to conceive. Some might call it a bad omen, yet dead birds often symbolize new beginnings and rebirth. But on this particular day, I lost it. I cried for the bird in my yard, I cried for my womb, I cried for my unborn baby. I cried as hard as I'd cried when I found out my dad had died. Uncontrollable tears exited my body and, looking back, I think perhaps my intense tears were also tears for the year and a half to come: the future hurt I would experience; the time I would spend waiting for my baby; and the baby I would lose along the way. That period feels so raw and vulnerable, but also necessary. That grief gave me the strength to carry on and eventually make it out the other side.

The path to surrender

I remember during our infertility process everyone would tell us we had to surrender, and I would think,

Okay, I'm going to surrender now. I would stand on my porch and look up at the sky and shout, "I SURRENDER! Now give me my baby." But surrender isn't something that you can force out of thin air; it's usually a place we are forced into. My moment of surrender came after we miscarried. I had finally gotten pregnant and I felt so proud, but when we found out the pregnancy wasn't viable, it truly hit me that I wasn't in control of my body. That's when I let go—not because I wanted to, but because there was no other option. I wasn't in charge; something much bigger than me was.

There is a fine line between surrender and giving up. In many ways they felt similar, but there were some key differences. When I surrendered, I internalized the truth that this wasn't in my hands or a choice I got to make. Maybe a baby would come again, and they wouldn't stay. Maybe we'd have to wait longer than we had dreamed of. Yet I was still doing everything I could to get pregnant: I went to doctors, started the process of IVF, took supplements, and continued to track my cycle. I didn't stop trying, but I did taper my expectations. I tried hard and I released control: a balancing act that took a long time to master. There was a breaking-down that happened, and that is how I managed to let go and accept my lack of control.

The way that we ended up pregnant is the story that I hated to hear when we were on our fertility journey. During our IVF round, there were a few hiccups which meant we had to take two months off. I was so mad that we had been delayed, but during that break, lo and behold, we got pregnant without any medical intervention. What happened to us plays into the narrative of "the second you stop trying, that's when it happens" and "all you need to do is relax and stop worrying." Every time I tell this story, someone says gleefully, "That's how it always happens!"

But I want to be clear: no, that is not how it always happens.

I don't want anyone else who is struggling to conceive, or feels otherwise betrayed by their body, to feel any more frustrated than they already are with being told to *relax*. I do not believe that when we give up control, suddenly everything we wish for just happens. Stories like mine are the stories we remember because they are more exciting than "it finally worked on our third embryo transfer." I didn't stop trying or stop worrying. I peed on ovulation sticks every morning, drove two hours every day to see my spouse who was working away from home; I controlled when and where and prayed to anything that would listen. I was not free as a bird, barefoot, and spontaneous. We got pregnant because it was our time to get pregnant. Simple as that.

Validate your worry

Coming to terms with the lack of control I have over my body has helped me with the anxieties that have accompanied my current pregnancy. Pregnancy after loss comes with its own set of challenges, and the fear of losing your baby becomes much more tangible once it's happened. I'm working to take some of what I learned during our infertility journey into this pregnancy. When we let go of specific expectations of how certain events will unfold in our lives, it can make it easier to accept when things don't go to plan. But it can also be scary to openly consider that things may not go how you want them to.

I used to believe that being open to non-optimal outcomes meant I was manifesting something bad to happen to me, by giving those thoughts energy. But I've learned that not worrying at all is not realistic for many of us, and that sometimes leaning into the worry can help you be prepared for all outcomes. By validating your worry but not letting it take over, you may find you feel more at peace with it.

I found the anxiety of the first trimester incredibly difficult. I was so scared to be happy because I worried any kind of celebration would make it harder if I miscarried. Then I felt mad, because I'd been waiting so long to get pregnant, and this anxiety was ruining the experience for me. The truth is, if I had miscarried, it would have been devastating. There is no way to sugarcoat that. But I would have gotten through it, like I had with my last miscarriage. That was what helped the most: knowing that if something bad happened, I would be able to handle it and plot out my next steps. I channeled my desire to control not into staying pregnant, which was not something I could control, but rather into my ability to deal with the aftermath. I love the way the book *Birthing from Within* by Pam England and Rob Horowitz talks about how worrying can sometimes be productive. They describe how worrying effectively can help shift frozen, fearful images of not being able to cope to more fluid images containing a variety of coping responses.

Drawing on these reserves to navigate my fertility journey has had broader implications in other areas of my life. Part of that is perhaps in relation to entering a new phase where I won't be able to control things in the way I'm used to. When it comes to work, I have had to accept that I'm not going to be able to look at every email or Instagram post that goes out when I have a baby. While I may still want to control that, I am also aware that there are other people around me whom I have to put my trust in, and that it's important for me to give them authority. Delegation can feel like surrender too. If I need to give up control of a project, I can feel better about it because I am empowering someone else in doing so. This has been a way for me to rationalize the release of control.

Appreciating where you can make an impact

Before we went through our fertility journey, I used to feel really responsible for all of the world's problems, and spent a lot of time feeling unhappy and hopeless that the world was messed up beyond repair. I'm not saying that we can't impact change, because people can and do make the world a better place in so many ways. But I took on so much responsibility in an attempt to control things that were completely out of my control, and this individual responsibility weighed me down in a way that wasn't healthy.

Today, I try to honor my desire to control life in a way that serves both me and others, rather than harming myself. We need to rewrite the narrative that we have the power to change every element of our existence if we are to build more compassionate and realistic expectations for ourselves. We need to work to let go of the myth that if only we had enough willpower or positive thoughts, the world would bend to our will. Many of the learnings I've shared in this chapter have meant that I've had to redraw the standards I hold myself to. I now accept that there are things I cannot overcome or steamroll over. Acknowledging that isn't an admission of failure, in the same way that giving up on the fight for control over uncontrollable forces isn't a sign of weakness. Adopting a neutral approach to all parts of our existence is an act of self-compassion, and an incredibly powerful one.

Do We Ever Really Get There?

Going into writing this book, I felt secure in my body neutral mindset. While I'd had my ups and downs, I believed my neutrality to be unshakable. I had a certain level of confidence that I'd "made it" close to the finish line. But when I got into the nitty-gritty of writing, I felt my body neutral mindset crumbling. Throughout the process of infertility, miscarriage, hormone injections, emotional distress, and then pregnancy—all of which occurred during the writing process—my body was the most in flux it's ever been. One day, I sat with my editor in near tears expressing that this was the least body neutral I had felt since I began healing from my eating disorders years ago. That's right—the body neutral author felt their least body neutral when writing the body neutral book. (Insert the applause emojis, because that is the most humbling ego-knockout ever.)

We are always students of neutrality, because humans are not designed to stay stagnant. We are ever-changing—fluid in our thoughts and feelings. We can't tick something off and assume it will never surface again. The challenges that arrive at our doors are a sign of being alive and existing in this world, and growth happens when we deal with them. Unlike when I was struggling with my eating disorder, this time I had a framework and a toolbox full of advice to draw from. The three steps which I outline in the book (acknowledge, explore, reconnect) supported me in so many ways. I would run through each of them in the morning in the shower and use them to pull myself out of the ditch. Did I instantly feel better? No. Did I have moments of frustration because I wanted to "fix" myself, and that wasn't happening? Yes. But I didn't summon old dangerous behaviors. In the middle of working on this book and having an existential crisis (because, yes, that is how it felt sometimes), something started to shift for me. I kept fighting the good fight, and every time it felt a little bit easier and a little bit clearer. After several weeks of this, I began to see the light and welcomed back the neutral mindset that had never really left me. Struggling with something doesn't make you a bad person and it doesn't mean you've failed: it helps you to move forward and get to the next place.

This experience has been a wonderful example that body neutrality isn't a destination; it's a practice that is sometimes easier and sometimes harder to implement. In hindsight, as I close this final chapter, I can see how the writing process has provided me with so much empathy for those who are first discovering body neutrality. It has reminded me how hard this journey can be, and that the path to healing is never linear. It has also reminded me that even when it feels like you're never going to get out of this cycle or that there is no hope, the things you've practiced and learned are still there to support you.

What writing this book has also underlined for me is how everything changes. When you feel stuck in a difficult moment, it's easy to believe that it's going to be that way forever. I'm here to remind you that isn't the case. Things constantly change and shift, sometimes for the better, sometimes for the worse, but one thing you can count on is that it won't be this way forever. That may feel uncertain, but I find a great deal of comfort in it too. Things will shift and I will shift with them. Neutrality has helped me to release expectations and stay open to all options and outcomes. I hope that, as you go forward, you too will see the lines that have been drawn for you and know you have the power to step outside of them. No matter what you have been taught about your body, your identity, or your aspirations, you are the one who gets to decide what you keep and what you leave behind.

One of the things that I have learned about myself in this long process of discovery is that I tend to find solace in extremes. I am most comfortable when I can put things in black and white, and it is really easy for me to attach to rigid ways of thinking. That is why I was enveloped by diet culture so deeply, and it's why I got caught up in toxic positivity too. The space in between, the rainbow, the neutral, is a huge challenge for me, because I was raised to believe there was only one way to be right and everything else was wrong. I still feel the pull to be all gung ho on one thing and believe in its absolute righteousness. There is comfort to be found in feeling like we are on the "right" side of any issue or way of life. The poles are attractive because they make us feel that we have a purpose, and that kind of validation is very difficult to walk away from.

While I continue to be attracted to extreme thinking, trends, and beliefs, and probably always will be, I'm now able to access the part of my brain that can put up a red flag and interrogate the situation before jumping in. Whenever I hear "This is the only way" or "You have to do this to get x, y, or z," especially when it comes to health and our bodies, I feel a jolt of recognition. It could be a clickbait headline—"This one drink will revolutionize the way you feel in the morning" (spoiler alert: lemon water is not going to solve all your problems)—or a product that promises to be a miracle superfood, or even a book advertised as the route to all happiness. Whatever it is, I go on red alert. It's natural to want the "easy answer," but with the exception of getting enough sleep and staying hydrated, there isn't something that is going to make every person feel better in their body. That's not to say I might not enjoy that book or superfood or lemon water. Maybe these things might complement what I'm already doing for myself and support me in a new way, but then maybe they won't. I can neutrally take in the information and stay curious, experiment and give it a try, while knowing that there's no magic wand for the hard stuff that life throws our way.

When you finish this book, I hope it's with a greater sense of curiosity. Being curious allows us to feel out all the different contours of our individual experiences, which is both exciting and deeply nourishing. The beauty of finding a more neutral approach is a sense of liberation. We are working to cast off the hard lines and boxes that other people have built around us. I would love to say that I don't care at all about what people think of me, but the people-pleaser in me will likely always struggle with that. However, I care far less than I once did, because I've allowed myself more room to play and more room to explore—which has brought with it more ways of living, thinking, and being. It is never too late to get curious and dabble in crossing the lines a little bit.

I also hope you finish this book with a heightened sense of awareness for when you're not being so kind to yourself, or when you're masking your feelings with toxic positivity, or when someone else is throwing a spanner in your body neutral work. I love it when people in my life tell me they had small *aha!* moments, like recognizing the instructor in their workout class is only talking about burning calories and not all the other benefits of movement. Or when they see those few extra pounds as something to be nurtured, not tortured. Or when they are unfazed by weigh-ins at the doctor, or unfollow that account that makes them feel bad about themselves. It's the little things that go the longest way. Cherish these moments!

In reading this book, you have already taken the first step. It may have been hard and challenging at times, and you may not have agreed with every single word in it, but I hope that as you turn the final page, you leave knowing that you are deserving. No matter who you are or what you look like, you are deserving of acceptance, deserving of love, deserving of food, joy, and community, deserving of respect. You are more than your body. I am more than my body. May we hold this awareness close as we navigate the world with a little more neutrality and a lot more love.

The Body Neutral Toolbox

Body neutrality is a constant journey, an ongoing practice, and something that can't be achieved with a snap of the fingers or a magic potion. It's work—rewarding work, but still work. The main chapters in this book are designed to give space to nuanced conversation and multiple experiences, while also acknowledging that it isn't easy! However, I also wanted there to be a place where you could immediately access a series of tangible tips that might support you on your body neutral journey—a stash of practical advice for the days when you need it most. I asked everyone I interviewed in the process of writing this book for their best tips, and here is a collection of their advice. Save your favorites and come back to them any time you need it.

Bethany says:

- **Ignore the tag.** When shopping for clothing, ignore the size on the tag and instead focus on how an item fits your body and how you feel in it. Giving your stomach space to expand, your lungs space to breathe, and your body more room to function can help you feel more comfortable and confident.

- **Stop labeling foods as "good" and "bad."** Food is food. It is not moral. Removing "good" and "bad" labels from food can help us be more neutral about the things we consume, which can lead to more well-rounded and stress-free meals.

- **Toss the scale.** I've said it once and I'll say it again. If the scale doesn't serve you, ditch it! Unless otherwise directed by your doctor or other health practitioner, there is no reason you need to know your weight. It is simply a measurement of your mass and not a measurement of your worth, happiness, or health.

- **Be kind to yourself.** I know this is easier said than done, but it really is an important reminder.

Inevitably, you're going to have easier days and you're going to have harder days. When the hard days come, be gentle with yourself. All of your feelings are valid and deserving of space, and not every feeling needs to be acted on. Meaning, let the feelings come and go without putting too much weight on them. Part of body neutrality is allowing space for the good stuff and the bad stuff while remembering that it's just stuff. YOU matter so much more than your body!

Alex says:

- **Knowledge is power.** Learning about the diet industry and why women in particular have such negative body image is so important and powerful.

- **Question your "why."** Engage critically with the pervasive thought that we need to be thinner. If you can't tap into the root of why you feel you need your body to be different to what it is, that in itself might give you the answers you need.

- **Set boundaries.** You can't force your learnings onto other people, but you can set boundaries to prioritize your mental health. That could look like sending a nice text explaining that you are on a journey to becoming comfortable in your body, and weight or diet talk isn't helping you right now. You are well within your rights to ask others to avoid those topics of conversation around you.

Alex Light (she/her) is a body confidence, self-acceptance, and lifestyle influencer from London. After struggling from various eating disorders, Alex transformed her virtual platform from a beauty and fashion blog into a glimpse into her personal struggles. Throughout her journey on social media, Alex has gained an expansive insight into the reality behind eating disorders, as well as weight stigma and diet culture. After a long and arduous recovery, Alex is dedicated to providing a safe space for anyone in the grips of an eating disorder or bad body image. Her bestselling book, *You Are Not a Before Picture*, is an urgent, enlightening, and empowering guide to disavowing diet culture and learning to make peace with our bodies.

Ally says:

- **Diversify your feed.** Get people with different identities and body sizes all over your Instagram and TikTok if you decide social media is a supportive space for you. If you find social media really tough, it's also okay to delete those apps or take a break.

- **Reframe statements into neutral ones.** If you're noticing yourself thinking things like *my stomach is too big*, practice reframing that in a neutral way. An example might be: *My stomach just is. This is who I am in this moment and I can't shift that. That is okay.* I find the act of saying it out loud is really important.

- **Try the mirror exercise.** This is something we use in our program. Look in the mirror naked, or in tighter clothes if that feels more comfortable, and list out fifteen positive or neutral comments about yourself. Exposing yourself to your body and getting used to the way that it looks and moves is vital.

Ally Duvall (she/her) is a fat activist and program manager at Equip Health, an eating disorder treatment program delivered at home. Ally's Substack, Fatpo-sially, speaks out against diet culture and anti-fat bias while uplifting fat joy. Ally grew up fighting a bru-tal eating disorder that went undiagnosed for several years. Medical providers missed the symptoms and focused solely on shrinking her body size. After start-ing treatment, she discovered her drive for fat activ-ism, health at every size, supporting others through recovery, and ensuring that fat folks are no longer excluded.

Chase says:

- **Lean on the people that you know care for you.** Not everybody is fortunate enough to come from families of origin that talk positively about weight, shape, size, and appearance. But sometimes you do have folks in your life who care deeply for you and nurture your well-being. Perhaps it's someone like a grandmother, or a great-aunt or a sibling or a best friend. Actively seek out time with those humans and allow their kindness to counterbalance the criticism from the outside world.

- **Let go of perfection.** When you are talking about body weight, shape, size, or appearance, sometimes the conversation is hard to have. A lot of folks are separating themselves from these topics because they worry they don't have the "perfect" thing to say. Remember that we are not going to get it right all the time, so allow yourself and others a little extra portion of grace.

Chase Bannister (he/him) is president of the board of the Eating Disorders Coalition for Research, Policy & Action, a licensed social worker, and CEO of Bannister Consultancy. He is a prominent figure in the architecture of mental health, recognized for his commitment and advocacy work in the field of treatment of eating disorders.

Cyrus says:

- **Remember that a thought is just a thought.** What does a thought really do? I step back and think, *What is this? Am I physically doing something right now?* No. It's me saying it to myself and I try not to give that thought power. That has helped me hugely.

- **Talk to your anxiety.** There is a makeup artist I know named Katy. I was on a trip with her one time, and we were talking about anxiety. Katy told me that when you are feeling anxious—about your appearance, or anything else—to talk to it. Challenge your anxiety as if it were a person, and dare it to make you feel worse. When you confront anxiety, it freezes up. It's a tactic that has changed my life.

- **Laugh at yourself.** Sometimes I laugh at myself, and comedy really does rebalance me. It helps me back to neutrality.

Cyrus Veyssi (they/he) is a creative strategist, DEI consultant, and digital creator. They are a seasoned content creator building intersectional digital spaces across the beauty and wellness world, and have been featured in *The Boston Globe, Allure, The Zoe Report, In the Know, Cosmopolitan*, and others. Cyrus is passionate about intersectional social issues, diversity and equity programming, social impact, innovative storytelling, and high fashion for all bodies. Cyrus is always working to challenge the gender binary and glass ceiling for queer professionals and emphasize inclusive workplace cultures.

Johanna says:

- **The ignorance stamp.** One of my favorite tools is called the ignorance stamp. Imagine that you have a rubber stamp with the word "ignorant" across it. When someone says something that is harmful or hurtful, imagine stamping their forehead. Then, as they continue to speak their harmful words, all you see is the word "ignorant." People are often not trying to be mean; they are just ignorant. I actually got some "ignorant" rubber stamps made up and I carry one in my purse!

- **Live in color.** Take a pack of crayons and pick a color to represent how you are feeling. When I started doing this, the only colors that felt safe were black and white because there was comfort in the binary. I gradually moved to an eight-pack of crayons, and over time made it to the sixty-four-pack. When I wasn't feeling good or bold, I would choose an ecru or a charcoal crayon. But doing this exercise reminded me that I deserve to live in the fuchsia or the chartreuse. That I had the chance to live in all those colors.

- **Look at how far you've come.** If you feel like you are moving backward, think back to where you've come from and where you are. It's a testament to yourself and your recovery to be able to give yourself that space and lean into it.

Johanna Kandel (she/her) is the founder and CEO of the National Alliance for Eating Disorders and an advocate, speaker, and the author of *Life Beyond Your Eating Disorder.* As a passionate advocate for mental health and eating disorders legislation, Johanna has spent a lot of time meeting with numerous members of Congress and was part of the first-ever Eating Disorder Roundtable at the White House. Johanna is a proud member of the Department of Health and Human Services's Interdepartmental Serious Mental Illness Coordinating Committee (ISMICC), is on the board of directors for the Eating Disorders Coalition, and is a member of the Eating Disorders Leadership Summit. She has received many awards for her ongoing outreach and advocacy work.

Lottie says:

- **Humor.** I think laughter and wit are always some of the greatest ways to find reconnection with yourself.

- **Social media.** For me (and this may be a divisive view!), using social media is a vital means of being creative, staying connected, and seeking involvement in community.

- **Writing.** Being expressive through writing is a great way to find empowerment and make sense of experiences.

- **Personal style.** Dressing up and playing with fashion is, for me, all about freedom and self-expression.

Lottie Jackson (she/her) is a writer, editor, and disability activist. Featured in *The Sunday Times Style*'s Women of the Year 2020 as "an important emerging voice," her work offers a vital dissection of the myths that beset disability. She has written for British *Vogue, Elle, The Guardian, The Sunday Times,* and *The Telegraph,* bringing her fresh perspective to the most urgent conversations of today about identity, social progress, and diversity. In 2020, she was selected for Penguin Random House's award-winning WriteNow program. Her writing redefines what it means to be disabled with nuance and wit, inspiring us to see new ways of existence. Her debut book, *See Me Rolling*, was published by Hutchinson Heinemann in 2023.

Megan says:

- **Eat with others.** They say that eating with your child is one of the most impactful things you can do. Even if you don't have kids, there is so much magic to eating with others. It reminds us that food is about so much more than nutrition. It's about connection, culture, memories, satisfaction, and sharing one of life's most simple pleasures with another person.

- **Keep your language neutral in front of children.** As the saying goes, if you can't say anything nice about your body in the mirror in front of your child, don't say anything at all. Or at least keep your language body neutral when you're talking about yourself in front of your child. You don't have to be a paragon of body neutrality, but try to not say negative things about yourself in front of young people.

Megan McNamee (she/her) is a registered dietitian nutritionist specializing in maternal/child nutrition and eating disorder prevention. She is the co-owner of Feeding Littles, which aims to empower families to raise adventurous, intuitive eaters. Megan holds a master's degree in public health nutrition and is a certified intuitive eating counselor.

Nina says:

- **Make the time for what centers you in your body.** Figure out what activities make you feel calmed, centered, or connected with your body. For me, it's movement like yoga, boxing, or swimming. For others, it's meditating, journaling, reading. Figure out what those things are, and carve out that time for yourself.

- **Find like-minded people to move with.** Finding friends or family who like doing the same types of activities as you is a great way to make movement about spending time together. And it can be more fun too!

- **Let go of comparisons when choosing activities.**
  Just because everyone is cycling or doing yoga doesn't
  mean you need to cycle or do yoga. Finding the activities that make you feel at home in your body doesn't
  always have to feel courageous or involve stepping
  outside of your comfort zone, and finding the ones
  you actually feel best doing will make them feel better!

Nina Kossoff (they/she) is a brand strategist whose passion lies in queer, transgender, and non-binary communities. Their career has spanned the music industry,
advertising, and health and wellness startups, always keep-
ing marginalized voices and well-being core to their work.
Nina led the proactive strategy at McCann that resulted
in Mastercard's True Name product allowing transgender
and non-binary people to put their chosen names on their
credit cards; and at FOLX Health they developed and
launched the HRT Care Fund to provide free access to
hormone replacement therapy to transgender and non-
binary Black and Indigenous people and people of color.
Nina is also the creator of ThemsHealth, an Instagram-
based resource for transgender and non-binary health and
wellness information, and an advisory council member

of Third Wave Fund, which resources and supports youth-led, intersectional gender justice activism.

Pooja says:

- **Shift from an external to an internal lens.** Say you decide to go to a yoga class because you have been told that it will support you physically and mentally. Are you gritting your teeth because you can't do a headstand and everyone else can? Or are you fully present and feel nourished afterward? You can do the same activity, but it can be a completely different experience depending on if your intention is external or internal. Don't be afraid to cast off those activities that don't nourish you internally.

- **Learn to recognize your anger.** Many of my patients don't recognize that they are angry about the world and how it has treated them. Admit that you are angry, and that it is okay to be angry. Then find containers for your anger—whether that's a therapist, a trusted friend, or a community—where you can express that anger with people who aren't scared of it, and discharge some of it in a nondestructive form. Releasing some of it will help you be less controlled by your anger.

- **Reflect before reacting.** So much of mental health and well-being comes from mentalization, which means you are able to reflect as opposed to simply reacting. You don't have to act on all of your feelings—you can feel them, move through them, and let them go. We know that people who build that capacity go on to have stronger mental health, and this is a framework that applies to so many decisions in life.

Dr. Pooja Lakshmin, MD, (she/her) is a psychiatrist, *New York Times* contributor, the author of *Real Self-Care*, and the founder and CEO of Gemma, the physician-led women's mental health platform. She is a leading voice at the intersection of mental health and gender, focused on challenging the tyranny of faux self-care. Pooja maintains an active private practice where she treats women struggling with burnout, perfectionism, and disillusionment, as well as clinical conditions like depression and anxiety. Having gone down the rabbit hole of extreme wellness herself, her book *Real Self-Care: A Transformative*

Program for Redefining Wellness (Crystals, Cleanses, and Bubble Baths Not Included) is her answer to the juice cleanses, the gratitude lists, and the bubble baths—not only to care for ourselves for real but, in turn, to transform our broken culture.

Stephanie says:

- **Walk around your house naked.** For a day or an evening a week. What a lot of us do when we look into the mirror, especially if we are naked, is we instantly pose and suck our stomachs in, turn to the side, or put one leg in front of the other to get that Barbic shape. Try to be naked and slouching. I find it such a great tool to seeing your body for what it is, and not something that needs to be fixed.

- **Take thirst traps**. It doesn't have to be for a partner—just for yourself. Buy underwear or things that make you feel sexy, strong, powerful, and confident. Then treasure those moments by taking a cute picture of yourself, to remember a time when you felt good, and know that that feeling will come around again.

- **Curate your social media.** Only follow accounts that spark joy. Maybe it's unfollowing the Kardashians or all these Instagram models, or brands that promote only one certain body type. Have the algorithm change so it shows more people and brands that look like you, and gradually your perception of what is normal will change.

Stephanie Yeboah (she/her) is a blogger, multi-award-winning content creator, author, host, freelance writer, public speaker, and body image/self-love advocate based in London. She also dedicates her time to advocacy within the body positivity, mental health, and self-love communities, sharing her own challenges and traumas involving fatphobia, bullying, self-esteem, and confidence issues, and the ways in which she's been able to turn it around while encouraging others to do the same. In 2020, she released her bestselling book *Fattily Ever After* and became the first British plus-sized Black woman to grace the cover of *Glamour* magazine.

Acknowledgments

Years ago I was in a large group setting where a medium was reading the crowd. Lo and behold, she started speaking to me. With sweaty palms I awaited what I would hear—messages from family members who have passed or untold stories that would change my life. But the medium only had one main message for me; she just kept saying, "Write! Journal! Put words on the page! There's a book in you!" I was surprised because while there was a tug in me that told me the prediction would be true, the idea of it actually happening was nothing short of terrifying. And yet somehow and someway, here I am putting the final words on the page of my very first book. There's a lot of people to thank.

The first is my editor, Anna. Without her we wouldn't have these pages at all. Thank you for taking what I always assumed would be a grueling experience and making it one of the most healing and important processes of my life. You truly have a gift.

To Katherine, my trusty cowriter who transcribed hours and hours of my thoughts, fears, tears, and stories to help organize and finesse them on the page. Thank you for creating a space where I could be open and vulnerable and show up as simply me.

To every voice who contributed to this book, I'm forever grateful. This book was never meant to be just my story. Your uniqueness and vulnerability have enhanced the pages, allowing so many others to see themselves within the words. Thank you thank you thank you to Alex Light, Ally Duvall, Chase Bannister, Cyrus Veyssi, Johanna Kandel, Lottie Jackson, Megan McNamee, Nina Kossoff, Pooja Lakshmin, and Stephanie Yeboah.

To Alexa, my business partner and friend, who knows how to reassure without bullshitting, motivate me when I'm defeated, and bring constant order to my constant chaos. Thank you for holding down the fort, excelling us forward and being the best Scorpio in all the land.

To my be.come clients. You all are the real stars. You often think that I teach you, but in reality you are the ones teaching me. I can't wait to continue to evolve together.

To Nico, the love of my life, father to my babies, and best friend in the world. You squashed every fear I had during this book writing process. I'm astounded by the capacity of our love, the strength of our bond, and the ability we have to constantly learn from one another. You make life a more beautiful place.

To Olive, our baby who never made it earth side, and to Kilmer Dove, our baby who is due in just a few weeks, the two of you have already taught me so much. You showed me the importance of grief and the sweetness of celebration. You challenged me, supported me, and encouraged me to keep fighting. You are woven into every line of this book and every beat of my heart.

To Cornerstone Press, Putnam, and the incredible Michelle Howry, thank you for believing in this book, taking a chance on me, and sharing the words found in this book with all of your readers. Forever grateful for the opportunity.

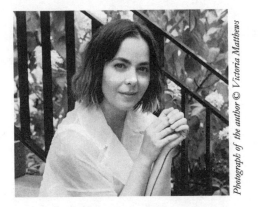

Photograph of the author © Victoria Matthews

Bethany C. Meyers (she/they) is the founder and CEO of the be.come project. She has been a part of the fitness industry for over fifteen years—as an instructor, a teacher trainer, and a workout creator. After battling an eating disorder for the majority of their fitness career, Bethany began to heal their relationship with exercise, food, and the physical self. Vowing to be the change she so desperately needed, Bethany founded the be.come project in July 2018, with the intention of sharing the powerful message of body neutrality with the world.

THEBECOMEPROJECT.COM

🐦 BethanyCMeyers
📷 BethanyCMeyers
📷 TheBecomeProject